The Persecuted Drug
The Story of DMSO

BY PAT MC GRADY, SR.

The Persecuted Drug: The Story of DMSO
The Savage Cell

The Persecuted Drug

The Story of DMSO

PAT McGRADY, SR.

Doubleday & Company, Inc.,   Garden City, New York
1973

ISBN: 0-385-08931-7
Library of Congress Catalog Card Number 73–79691
Copyright © 1973 by Pat McGrady, Sr.
All Rights Reserved
Printed in the United States of America
First Edition

TO GRACE—for her literary suggestions, and

TO MANY FRIENDS IN SCIENCE, MEDICINE AND
GOVERNMENT—for their considerable help in gathering
and interpreting a mountain of material,

This book is gratefully and affectionately dedicated.

Foreword

My editor, Larry Ashmead, wanted a nice, simple, straightforward book about a strange chemical called DMSO, or, formally, dimethyl sulfoxide. Something, he said, about the compound's unusual chemical and physical properties. And, to be sure, something about the unrestrained claims made for its healing powers. Something factual, reasonable, sound.

I was delighted. There was nothing I would rather write than a nice, simple, straightforward book about DMSO, whose fortunes I had followed closely for years. I reviewed the bushels of notes, reprints, correspondence, news stories, and other materials; and it was evident at once that my problem was not a paucity of evidence but a proliferation of scientific and medical data. Boiling it all down to publishable—and, hopefully, palatable—size and form would call for an effort of major magnitude. And, on further contemplation, it became evident that the quantity element was subordinate to the quality factor; to anyone familiar with the medical scene, the facts about DMSO seemed like sheer fantasy.

Even if DMSO were a snake oil, a nostrum, a remedy promoted by a band of quacks, there might be an entertaining story about charlatans, the credulous public and the protection afforded by a watchful government and a concerned medical profession. The weakness in this thesis lay in the readily demonstrable fact that

vii

the academic and professional credentials of those espousing DMSO were, by and large, superior to those of the challengers. And, it was very clear, the scientists and physicians who championed DMSO were doing so on the basis of their experience with the drug; most of the critics had never seen, touched, or—and this is important—even smelled it.

Assuming that this text could be supported adequately, one would be confronted by the embarrassingly logical question: If DMSO is that good, why isn't it on every drugstore shelf in America? The answer to this question can be summed up in a single word—bureaucracy. And if that answer is as unsubstantial for the reader as it would be for this writer, one might add, by way of explanation and amplification: Read the exposé by James S. Turner and other "Nader's Raiders" (*The Chemical Feast*), the remarkably candid confessions by federal government committees, the Kinslow Committee report and the Ritts Committee report, the admissions by high government officials, usually after abdicating, and testimony by countless other qualified authorities.

The question then arises: If bureaucracy is as it is described by these eminent authorities, how could DMSO—or any new drug—ever survive? The answer is: Because the scientist who discovered its therapeutic potential is a person who just did not understand intimidation and fear, dissembling and cheating, money and the other materialistic rewards which govern lives and systems.

So, as it turns out, the purchaser of this book gets not a single, simple, straightforward account of a drug but three stories in one: the incredible performance of an unbelievable drug; the unlikely adventures of a fantastic government agency; and the problems of a man so good in a wicked world that his virtues are regarded as vices.

Sorry, Larry.

Part One

This is the story of a drug which was glorified briefly as having almost panacean properties for the ailments of man and beast and diseases of plant life and then was banished by high United States Government authorities as dangerous and without merit.

This is also the story of a mild-mannered scientist who challenged the law and defied the officials and their police in a soul-searing struggle to make the drug available wherever there is life.

The drug is known as DMSO, or dimethyl sulfoxide. It has been championed by reputable physicians as capable of healing or palliating many ailments. It has been represented as a "wonder drug" or a "miracle drug." It is abundant; it can be extracted from such sources as coal, oil or, most commonly, lignin, the material nature uses to cement cells together in trees; it is cheap; it is most often administered by simply dabbing it on the skin; and, alone or as a carrier for other drugs, which DMSO often potentiates, it penetrates the skin to enter the bloodstream and be borne to all parts of the body.

Most doctors and the public remember DMSO as a sort of cure-all that was found to be terribly toxic—like thalidomide. This allegation is perpetuated in periodic "white papers" distributed by the FDA—the Food and Drug Administration—the agency of the Department of Health, Education, and Welfare charged with protecting America's physical and mental well-being against the ever present hazards of dangerous drugs, foods, appliances and cosmetics.

The white paper, "Chronology of Dimethyl Sulfoxide (DMSO)," totaling as many as thirty-five pages, has given no indication whatsoever that DMSO has benefited any animal or human. It alludes to unidentified "reports" of severe harm to patients on DMSO therapy with some of the side effects, like anaphylactic shock, potentially lethal. Emphasis on damage to organs in laboratory animals given DMSO implies that the drug could be deadly to man.

Scientists contend that the thousand and more papers published in professional journals refute virtually all the FDA's charges. They state that in every instance of severe animal toxicity, DMSO had been administered in enormous quantities, usually by bizarre routes, and sometimes to establish the lethal dose.

The prosecution of DMSO and its defense, as reported here, are based upon ten years of extensive investigation, careful study of all the available literature, interviews with some top Food and Drug Administration officials, visits with patients, talks with physicians, and observation at two large international scientific conferences on DMSO. My family, friends and I have used DMSO for a variety of complaints.

The year was 1866. The place was Kazan, even then an important city on the Volga River in Central Russia.

Dr. Alexander M. Saytzeff held a test tube up to the light and examined its contents. The stuff looked like water; it was colorless and clear; it had a barely perceptible scent of sulfur about it. He may have put a drop or two on a glass rod and tasted it; it was slightly bitter and left an oysterish aftertaste and odor. His fingers felt it; it was a little viscous—not much. But decidedly there was something odd about it; it left the skin warm—almost hot; it had a drying effect on the tissues. He identified it as DMSO, or dimethyl sulfoxide.

4

Strangest of all was its avidity for other substances. It dissolved almost everything he added to it. Saytzeff put the fluid on his shelf, took it down occasionally to test its unusual physical and chemical qualities, and wrote a little article on its synthesis which appeared in 1867 in a journal published in Germany.

Saytzeff eventually went to his grave and his discovery, to all intents and purposes, was buried with him. For eighty or ninety years, it served as little more than as a conversation piece among chemists.

DMSO is a small and simple molecule, especially when one considers the impressive spectrum of its effects upon living and non-living matter—a versatility possibly unequaled by any other chemical designed by God or man.

$$
\begin{array}{c}
O \\
\| \\
S \\
\text{II-C-II II-C-II} \\
\text{| |} \\
\text{H } \text{ H}
\end{array}
$$

It is composed of two methyl (CH_3) groups and a sulfur and an oxygen atom, all of them stacked up in the shape of a pyramid. The sulfur pole has a strong negative charge, and the oxygen a positive charge, and the resulting electromagnetic-type force enables one DMSO molecule to attach to another—negative pole to positive pole—and form molecular chains.

For eighty years, scientists did not go far beyond Saytzeff's rudimentary findings. Then, gradually, in scattered laboratories around the world, researchers started mounting investigations of its curious capabilities. The fact that DMSO began to have commercial value in a few industries made the research rewarding enough.

Some of the inquiry delved into the structure of DMSO itself —a molecular Gibraltar able to resist formidable forces which would swallow it, shatter it or in some way change it. It had sturdiness to spare; it stabilized neighboring compounds and even entire structures in living cells.

DMSO was found to be unique in its promiscuous embrace of other molecules, in the strength of its bonds, its imperviousness to cold, its striking propensity for giving off heat and for undoing the effect of radiations, its ghostlike ability to penetrate tissue and cell walls and to transport other substances with it. In probably unparalleled chemical compatibility, DMSO was shown to mix readily with other solvents—water, alcohol, oils (lipids) and benzene among them.

Some research was of a fundamental nature—as they say, to develop knowledge solely for the sake of knowledge. Other studies were practical—to produce a better synthetic fiber or an improved solvent for resins, dyes, paints, or agricultural chemicals. DMSO production by United States pulp and paper mills began to mount sharply in the mid-1950's because of the solvent's increasing utility in various industries; by the mid-1960's, it had gone from a few thousand pounds a year to five million. The big stimulus stemmed from optimistic reports of DMSO's role in medicine.

The highly technical chemical data suggested to imaginative scientists a diverse therapeutic potential for DMSO.

DMSO freezes at about room temperature (a little more than 18° C or 68° F) and boils at a similarly high temperature (189° C or 372° F). Because it combines with water, it reduces ice-crystal formation. With this clue, British scientists discovered that DMSO was a gentle and effective coolant which permitted the storage of blood cells and their source, bone marrow. Even at 50° C below zero a 50 per cent mixture of DMSO and water will not freeze.

DMSO's abilities, at various concentrations, to donate protons to other molecules and to trap charged flying atoms and clusters of atoms (free radicals, so-called) permit it to maintain order amid the chaos of the dynamic micro-world of inner space. This suggested that DMSO might undo or prevent radiation damage to living systems.

6

DMSO has a great capacity to dehumidify locally by sopping water out of the environment. It gets rid of the water shell around many substances and then dissolves them—that is, it floods into the spaces between the solute molecules, delicately separating and suspending them. It does this for simple gases, resins (in some lacquers), sugars, cellulose derivatives and dextran, the blood plasma expander.

It also alters some antibiotics and the basic components of living matter—proteins and nucleic acids. This finding made DMSO a candidate for testing as a potentiator of preparations for disease control in humans, animals and plants.

In high concentrations, DMSO denatures, or demolishes, the basic chemical components of life, nucleic acids and some proteins; it breaks them up so they can never be put together again. In low concentrations, DMSO may gently dissolve the same proteins and activate them. This dual influence on the proteins would endow DMSO with a vast potential of enzymatic effects. Enzymes are proteins which catalyze the many thousands of reactions in the body's essential chemistry. By activating or inhibiting various enzyme systems, DMSO presumably turns on and off various physical and mental functions. It is possible, for example, that by suppressing the enzyme cholinesterase, which catalyzes certain reactions in the C fibers of nerves, DMSO might block the chemical pathway transmitting the pain sensation. Or DMSO might dissolve or denature a virus's protein coat of armor and leave the viral nucleic acid core, should it survive the DMSO onslaught, naked, defenseless and subject to attack by the host's immune arsenal. Some believe that this and any of several other properties might also sterilize or kill bacteria and fungi.

The simple solvent gradually has acquired a long and varied repertoire of other reactive talents on which an imaginative scientist could hypothesize numerous medical applications. DMSO's ability to chelate, or claw, certain metals out of molecules recommends it, theoretically, for a gamut of uses, from treating lead poisoning to correcting certain inherited disorders; it now

7

is known to dissolve and partially detoxify some poorly absorbed quaternary ammonium salts. Its stabilizing effect on some of the cell's sources of ready-made enzymes (mitochrondria and lysosomes), its harmless handling of enzymes, its power to dissolve a great many essential body chemicals—fatty acids, sterols, polysaccharides, and the like—suggest that the uses of DMSO may be limitless. One research group has used DMSO to extract edible keratin proteins from goose feathers.

Investigators in widely scattered parts of the world have reported on the curious physical and chemical attributes of DMSO: Austrians on the molecule's Raman spectra and polarization data, Scandinavians on its structure, Americans on its vapor pressure and thermodynamic properties, Canadians on its association with water, Finns on its behavior when mixed with benzene, Germans on its solvent abilities, Japanese on its use in synthetic manufacturing, and the British on DMSO's protection against damage by cold.

It was this last bit of information that climaxed a young American surgeon's search and projected him from the quiet of his ivory tower into a life of high adventure.

It was a large room on the sixth floor of the University of Oregon Medical School complex. It was brightly lighted, utilitarian, smelling of non-fragrant chemicals, and noisy with the clink of glassware, the splash of water in the large sink, the clatter of a typewriter, and the supersonic sensations emanating from laboratory machines.

A few young men and women worked at the long glass-strewn table. A secretary typed industriously at an orderly desk.

Two men were deep in conversation at a desk cluttered with journals, notepaper, records of various dimensions and a small stack of manuscripts.

The smaller man in the white coat, the surgeon, watched in fascination as the man in the brown suit, the chemist, rubbed India ink on a twig and then applied a colorless fluid to it. The fluid seemed to drive the ink into the twig.

"It does that with antibiotics too," the chemist said.

"How about human tissues?" the surgeon asked.

The chemist said, "It seems to penetrate to the deeper layers of the skin. A dermatologist at Stanford once told me that if it did that, they might have to rewrite the dermatology textbooks."

The episode, late in 1961, was to change the surgeon's life drastically. And the chemist's life. And the destinies of many others as well.

The chemist was Robert J. Herschler, who bore the title Supervisor, Applications Research, Chemical Products Division, Crown Zellerbach Corp., Camas, Washington. CZ is one of the biggest pulp and paper manufacturers in the world. Camas is across the bridge from Portland and a half-hour's drive up the Columbia River.

The surgeon was Stanley Wallace Jacob, M.D., F.A.C.S., Assistant Professor of Surgery, University of Oregon Medical School.

Both men were thirty-seven years old. Herschler, a six-footer weighing 180–90 pounds, was five inches taller and thirty pounds heavier than Jacob. In their professions, their aptitudes, their life modes, their social and academic backgrounds, they were far apart. But in one thing—their complete zeal for and dedication to the watery stuff they were examining—they became identical twins.

Herschler was the hard-working son of hard-working parents. He paid much of his own way through high school in the state of Washington and through Washington University in St. Louis, Missouri, where he received his highest academic award—a Bachelor of Science degree. Soon after graduation, he got a job with Crown, and for twenty-odd years he had been a faithful—albeit often unhappy—employee of that concern.

With only a Bachelor of Science degree but endowed with considerable aptitude for chemistry and a nagging curiosity about biological phenomena, Herschler resided in an academic, cultural, and economic twilight zone reserved for over-qualified non-doctors. One of a familiar breed of talented untouchables in a degree-conscious community, Herschler was outranked in his firm by men he felt were less competent. He was a creature of an industrial colossus, he said, bound by unuttered vows of humility, obedience and silence. He was paid the wage which good—but non-doctoral—chemists command in a small town setting, and, with this and his wife's salary as a teacher, he had built a good home with his own hands and maintained his family of three daughters in comfort. He reacted as any man does to orders which he considered less than reasonable; but he did what was required and held his job.

What hurt most, Herschler complained, was the silence imposed on him. It was not that the professional caste system carries a good deal of weight with doctor-conscious journal editors, it was the rigid censorship imposed by industry. Scientific data and ideas are treated in industry generally as trade secrets; and they are mentioned abroad only with the firm's consent—and usually to advance commercial ends. The chemist was exploding with ideas that needed uttering.

For more than a year Herschler had been seeking one of the academic elite—an M.D. or a Ph.D.—to discuss the interesting compounds he had teased out of trees as they were converted into newsprint and toilet tissue. One of the chemicals was DMSO. There were others which he felt might be of value in science or medicine.

For many months, Dr. Stanley W. Jacob had been seeking a way to cool his isolated dog hearts. He had stored the living organs under enormous pressures; he had tried a succession of antifreeze chemicals. Nothing stopped ice crystals from forming and killing the delicate cells.

When the British reported success with DMSO as a preservative for blood and marrow cells, he devoured every word he could find on the chemical and physical properties of DMSO. And now across the table sat a man who knew—and had—DMSO, a whole gallon container of it.

Unlike Herschler, Jacob had been blessed in abundance with the professional privileges, the triumphs and the trophies that the chemist had been denied. He was a Fellow of the American College of Surgeons, an Assistant (soon to be Associate) Professor of Surgery in a department headed up by the prestigious Dr. J. Englebert Dunphy. He had held the emblem of all-around intellectual excellence, a five-year Markle Scholarship in Medical Sciences, an honor bestowed on those with towering IQ's. Customarily he had been at the top of his class, or very close to

11

it, in grade school in Atlantic City, N.J., and high school in Youngstown, Ohio. During his undergraduate years at Ohio State University, as a science major, he ranked first in his premedical class; he had his B.A. at age twenty-one and his M.D. (cum laude) at twenty-four—in 1948, the year Herschler got a job with Crown. He completed his internship, residency, and a three-year research fellowship at Harvard Medical School and its teaching hospitals and became the chief resident in surgery under Dunphy at Harvard's big and busy Boston City Hospital.

Herschler, his friends said, was a quiet, sober, sensitive, introspective sort. The fires of enthusiasm were great but they burned inside him—where they could not be quenched by what he felt were socially superior but intellectually superficial materialists about him.

Jacob, on the other hand, was outgoing. In high school he was a cheerleader, and a Ping-Pong champion, senior class president, state champion in oratory and in debate. He was a member of a dozen scholarly and professional organizations, including Phi Beta Kappa, and Alpha Omega Alpha (the upper ten percentile, nationally). He had won such honors as the Kemper Foundation Research Scholarship of the American College of Surgeons (1957–60) and First Place Glycerine Research Award, 1959. He was a lieutenant colonel in the U. S. Army Medical Corps Reserve and had served in Japan during the Korean War. He had published more than forty papers in scientific journals on such research as overcoming surgical shock, the prophylactic use of antibiotics, and the problem of restoring blood production in leukemic children treated with lethal doses of radiation. (He was successful in restarting blood cell synthesis in lethally irradiated dogs by inserting a marrow-producing healthy rib into their spleens.)

At the time of his meeting with Herschler, Jacob was seeking a means of cooling viable organs from freshly dead donors; his idea was to preserve the hearts so that, when needed, they could be taken out of cold storage and grafted into the recipient at once; this would replace the ghoulish practice of pacing the floor impatiently, waiting for the donor to die—or, worse, speeding his demise. Even at this early date, 1961, when heart transplants were discussed mainly in science fiction, Jacob and his team were making puppy hearts beat in adult dogs for several days at a time.

On this early winter afternoon, Herschler told Jacob of the day when DMSO solutions of basic dyes had been spilled accidentally; the color seemed to seep into deeper areas of the skin of workmen who had been splashed. When a DMSO solution of pesticidal DDT was spilled, those who were in the way became sick. Herschler told how DMSO solutions of antibiotics and antifungal agents had penetrated the surface of plants, and he surmised that DMSO might have a valuable place in treating plant diseases.

Late that evening, before he closed his lab, Jacob applied iodine to his arm, dabbed DMSO over the spot, and sat there watching the iodine disappear into the deeper regions of the skin. As he watched, he suddenly became aware of a strange thing: He could taste the DMSO! This meant that DMSO not only went deep into the skin but actually went through the skin, into the bloodstream and throughout the system!

The young surgeon rose to his feet and paced the floor, a thousand ideas clamoring for recognition. Did DMSO open a new door from the outer environment into the body? Would DMSO serve as a train to transport drugs through the skin to the internal organs? Could it be that DMSO represented not merely a new drug but an entire new principle in the treatment of disease?

Jacob did not sleep well that cold night. He hasn't slept very well ever since. Visions held siege in the brain regions meant for dreams.

The next day Jacob applied DMSO to the backs of the hands of his lab staff. Most of them reported the oysterish taste; the odor came quickly onto the breath of every one of them.

And some said the DMSO seemed to have a drying effect on the skin where it had been dabbed on. It occurred to Jacob that if this were so, DMSO applied to skin burns might prevent infections in the moist areas under scabs, a common and sometimes serious complication. He and Herschler set up a little experiment in which eighteen rats, under anesthesia, received scald burns on the back. The six treated with DMSO were much quieter and presumably more comfortable than the six treated with salt solution and the other six given no treatment.

The experiment had little if any scientific significance; but a little later, when Herschler sustained a chemical burn on his hands, forearms and forehead, DMSO was applied; the pain subsided in five minutes and stayed away for four hours, when a second application of DMSO again dispelled it.

When one of Herschler's assistants sprained an ankle, DMSO was applied liberally; the pain was relieved in fifteen minutes and the swelling in a half-hour.

An arthritic thumb was painted with DMSO, and in less than an hour pain and swelling were reduced.

Clinical experiments of this sort—each could be described as a "series of one case"—don't constitute scientific proof of anything. They did convince Jacob, however, that DMSO demanded urgent attention. He moved impulsively to seek new biological activities in the watery stuff. He worked tirelessly to confirm his observations in animals, then in humans—first of all, on himself.

Jacob rapidly came to recognize in DMSO not only its ability to pass into the skin carrying other substances with it, but he found further that DMSO would deposit many of these materials in the bloodstream, that it would pass through otherwise impenetrable membranes, that alone it possessed dramatic healing properties, and in combination with certain other drugs, it exercised an additive or multiplying effect.

For him, his long workday now became much too brief. Dawn came too late; night—when wearily he would turn out the light in his lab and leave a deserted building and cross a silent campus —fell too soon.

As DMSO bared its chemical and biological secrets to him, one by one, Jacob became convinced that the strange tree juice offered the art and science of medicine a boon of major magnitude.

Convincing others was to be another matter.

It was not entirely by accident that Jacob happened to have DMSO with him on those numerous occasions when someone needed it. After testing the drug on himself with enormous doses and on willing associates with smaller—but still large—doses, the young surgeon carried a bottle of the drug in his coat pocket wherever he went.

On Army Reserve training, an enlisted man—a football player for Portland State College—told Jacob that he had a splitting headache and asked to be excused from a half-mile run. Jacob showed him some DMSO, told him a little about its properties, and asked if the enlisted man would mind if he dabbed a little on his forehead. The headache cleared up within minutes, and the man ran the half-mile. The headache returned after four hours and once again was suppressed with DMSO.

The chief nurse at a county hospital had Jacob apply DMSO to a painful cold sore on her upper lip. When she called him on the telephone a couple of hours later, Jacob said expectantly, "Dorothy, you're going to tell me that the DMSO dried up your cold sore and it's going away?"

"No," Dorothy said. "It's better than that. It cleared up a sinusitis I've been fighting without any luck. For the first time in three months I'm breathing normally and easily through that nasal passage."

15

For Jacob, life was becoming full of serendipity—surprise discoveries, unexpected revelations, unsought disclosures.

There was the day an intern called Jacob's attention to Daisy, a skinny little six-year-old who for three years had lived in pain. She had rheumatoid arthritis in her neck and hip. On this occasion Jacob petted her out of her low-moaning misery and asked, "Honey, do you mind if I rub a little of this stuff where it hurts?" Because everything long ago had lost the power to assuage the pain, Daisy wasn't too keen about the idea, but finally she gave in. A half-hour later, the little girl turned her head and moved her shoulder. She hadn't been able to do that in two years.

After a good deal of coaxing, Daisy finally let herself be lifted from her crib; and, clinging to the surgeon's elbow with matchstick arms, she tottered on her wasted legs. Then, unsupported, she walked a few steps alone.

Daisy bawled. When the doctor asked why she was crying, Daisy said happily, "Because it doesn't hurt any more."

There were failures, of course. Failures galore. The dose that seemed to work for one patient had no effect at all in another with an apparently identical condition.

And, Jacob knew, any of the individuals he had treated successfully quite conceivably could have been helped by a placebo effect. A placebo (from the Latin meaning "I shall please") is a sugar pill, or an injection of distilled water, or a teaspoonful of an innocuous (but preferably bitter-tasting) fluid. Somewhere between 20 and 50 per cent of cancer patients given a placebo will report feeling better, and a few of them may gain weight, eat better, sleep well or show other objective signs of improvement—for a while.

There was no way of telling for sure whether DMSO had exerted a true physiological effect or served as a psychological crutch in almost any of the patients Jacob treated. One would be naïve not to suspect that a placebo effect was involved in any one case of the instant clearing of headaches, the immediate improvement in arthritics, or any of the numerous other "miracles" that followed dabbing DMSO on the skin. At the same time, one would have to be a simpleton to attribute all the remarkable effects solely to placebo properties.

Because, by and large, animals are less suggestible and therefore superior to humans as experimental subjects, Jacob and his associates ran countless laboratory experiments. It was expedient, for example, to learn in the lab whether DMSO would prevent adhesions from forming following certain surgical procedures. At least there would be minimal emotional effects involved in efforts to keep organs in the rat belly from sticking together or to the wound following a sham operation. Dilute (15 per cent) DMSO was instilled into the body cavities of one half the operated rats for ten days after surgery; nothing was done for the other rats. At the end of the experiment, the animals were opened up and examined. Results: completely negative. There were just as many adhesions in the DMSO-treated rodents as in the controls.

Jacob mulled it over for a few days and wondered what role the timing had played. He repeated the experiment with one change: he administered the DMSO before surgery, rather than after it. Result: DMSO greatly reduced the number of adhesions.

It appeared that DMSO could suppress inflammation—a benefactive potential for both patient and doctor in countless life-threatening and other worrisome situations.

DMSO was cheap—it could be produced for thirty-five cents a pint, and a pint represented, on the average, a month's generous supply for most large households. Moreover, it could be produced in any quantity, pretty much as a runoff product of the pulp and paper industry. "I could pipe it down here for you," Herschler once told Jacob. "You could have it by the barrel or the tank."

Research, even on animals, is costly, however, and it soon became necessary for Jacob to scratch for financial support well beyond the funds he could spare from his own salary. Some dealers in laboratory supplies were beginning to show impatience over past-due bills.

Jacob finally decided to appeal to his dean, Dr. David W. E. Baird.

Baird, who later retired, was regarded as an intelligent and charismatic head of the University of Oregon Medical School faculty. He encouraged creative ideas among those capable of developing them; he abided by principles of decent and tolerant human conduct for himself and sternly forbade any and all under his dominion from abridging the rights of others; he was bluff, amiable, sensitive to the needs and weaknesses of others, but, withal, a no-nonsense man.

Dean Baird listened attentively to the young surgeon, who had dressed for the occasion in a correct Ivy League-type suit, with manners to match. Jacob told the head of the school hierarchy how he became interested in DMSO, what he had done with it so far, and the role he hoped it would play in medicine.

"The trouble is," Jacob said, "I've diverted into this work all I can spare."

He paused for a long minute, as the older man leaned back in his swivel chair and studied him carefully. The dean had heard about DMSO; some of the reports and rumors had been carried to him as complaints from faculty members who neither relished Jacob's unrestrained enthusiasm for the drug nor approved his swashbuckling trials on a large number of unrelated pathological conditions. Some faculty members would be most unhappy if Jacob were encouraged. Nevertheless, when at length Dean Baird spoke, he said, "I think that the university might be able to spare a little support for something as promising as DMSO. Would five thousand dollars help?"

It would. And it did. Jacob had found a powerful benefactor.

The fortunes of DMSO were governed by the vagaries of chance in areas completely unrelated to the compound's role in science and medicine.

These factors were first interjected into the DMSO story—without anyone's being aware of the fact—on the morning of March 13, 1962, at a seminar for science writers in the Ramada Inn in odoriferous proximity to the slaughterhouse in San Diego, California.

George E. Moore, M.D., Ph.D., F.A.C.S., who had rebuilt the nondescript Roswell Park Memorial Institute of Buffalo, N.Y., into one of the world's most productive research centers, began his lecture by walking to the blackboard and writing in large block letters:

T-H-A-L-I-D-O-M-I-D-E

"Note that name well," he told the writers. "You'll be reporting it for some time to come."

Thalidomide was a drug produced in Germany—the perfect sedative, some have called it. It was said to have no aftereffects.

"What we have not been told is that thalidomide damages the unborn," Moore said. "Dr. Helen B. Taussig of Baltimore returned recently from Europe with information that between three and four thousand malformed babies have been born to German

19

mothers who had been taking thalidomide during their pregnancies; between one and two thousand additional cases have occurred in the United Kingdom."

Moore talked about cancer research at Roswell Park and then, already overdue for conferences at home, he headed for the airport and nosed his own plane toward winter and Buffalo.

Without opportunity to question Moore fully, only two of the writers mentioned thalidomide, and these references were brief and buried deep in their stories.

Four months later the story broke out of Washington—the FDA announcement commanded screaming eight-column bannerlines and page one play. Dr. Taussig said at the time, "We should be grateful the drug was not dreamed up in this country. It could have passed the Food and Drug Administration under our present laws."

President Kennedy a month or so after the news break pinned a medal on Dr. Frances O. Kelsey of the FDA for her heroic passivity in not favoring thalidomide in the long backlog of new drugs awaiting FDA approval. Inasmuch as thalidomide was not introduced abroad until 1958 and it was taken off the market late in 1961, Kelsey may not have had to exercise much restraint to save American embryos from phocomelia, the congenital deformity. The situation was not without a happy side: the story and picture of President Kennedy decorating Kelsey made page one and warmed the hearts of all good Americans, especially those in the FDA's corps of press agents.

Among those who heard Moore's brief account of thalidomide effects was Dr. Stanley W. Jacob of the University of Oregon, another speaker. He had not the slightest inkling at this time that thalidomide would play a crucial role in shaping his career.

Jacob the next day delivered a lively and scholarly dissertation—twenty-four pages of observations on his and his associates' attempts to preserve human spermatozoa, dog and rabbit skin, conjunctival cells and tissues by cooling them to temperatures as low as minus $272.2°$ C and a score of other studies.

Jacob did not mention DMSO on this occasion. He had only begun serious studies with it.

Joan F. Giambalvo, M.D., of the FDA once drew up a chronology of the misery on which her agency had thrived prior to the thalidomide incident.

It took the deaths of ten children from diphtheria antitoxin contaminated with tetanus to impel Congress to pass the Virus, Serum and Toxin Act of 1902, the nation's first effort to regulate drug manufacturing. The existing law (of 1848) merely had prohibited the importation of adulterated drugs—a statute offering obvious advantages for American pharmaceutical houses.

The 1906 Pure Food and Drug Act was a consequence of Upton Sinclair's *The Jungle*, a stomach-turning account of meat-packing practices. At the same time, Dr. Harvey W. Wiley's "poison squad" of young U. S. Department of Agriculture employees exposed the incorporation of dangerous additives in food.

Additional restrictions were imposed after finding cataracts in more than 100 people who took dinitrophenol to reduce the mysterious female illnesses which finally were traced to thallium in a depilatory, and then, in 1937, the death of more than 100 people from Elixir of Sulfanilamide containing a highly toxic solvent, diethylene glycol. Congress reacted in 1938 by requiring that new drugs pass safety tests and that the data be submitted to the government for clearance. The 1938 law, while tending to assure the safety of drugs, did nothing to require their efficacy. Worthless preparations could be peddled freely so long as they were harmless.

Then came thalidomide.

In August of 1962, the proposed new FDA regulations were published for comment. They had been discussed for years, but the teratogenic horror that swept over Germany and the United Kingdom made American action mandatory and urgent. Congress pressed the panic button.

The Kefauver-Harris Amendments called for extensive and expensive protocols in the basic testing of drugs—so expensive, in fact, that millions of dollars had to be poured into any drug's being tested, and so time-consuming they were unworkable in a bureau already years behind schedule. The FDA was given police powers like those exercised by gang-busting agencies; they called for intricate divisions and subdivisions of an organization already so intricately divided and subdivided and duplicative that it was unmanageable; they spawned a whole new lexicon of legalistic definitions and jargonistic initials. They introduced chaos where there had been only confusion.

If aspirin were to be submitted today for FDA approval the producer would have to submit to considerable preliminary investigations and three phases of testing before he could market his drug. Some authorities say that under current regulations aspirin would never make it to the drugstore counter.

First of all, the producer would have to apply for an IND (Investigational New Drug Exemption) permit from one of the many FDA bureaus (heart and kidney, metabolism and hormone, cancer and radiation drugs, nerves, dental, anti-infection, etc.). Because aspirin is used in something like thirty-eight fairly well defined situations, a good deal of time would be spent determining which and how many bureaus would have jurisdiction over the testing. The filing in triplicate of an IND usually qualifies the drug to be shipped (for laboratory studies) in interstate commerce.

Aspirin undoubtedly would be denied the privileges that go with filing of an IND; its widespread prior use as a cure-all for headaches, rheumatoid arthritis and many other conditions would have put it in what the FDA calls a controversial status—along with hallucinogenic LSD and panacean DMSO, the two taboos of the 1960–70's.

If aspirin eventually received the blessings of three men from each of the bureaus—a medical FDA officer, pharmacologist and chemist—permission to test aspirin in humans could reasonably be expected. Chances are the FDA would be aghast at the lack of controlled studies in animals and humans, however, and it would withhold permission.

Highly trained clinical pharmacologists, armed with bushels of data accumulated in test-tube and animal studies, would then seek to trace any deleterious effects aspirin might have had on humans. They and the doctors who aided them could determine the toxic effects on organs and systems, how it is metabolized, absorbed and eliminated, what happens to it after various routes of administration (by mouth, vein, artery, etc.), safe dosage, and the like.

If aspirin passed inspection by one or a few pharmacologists, it would be graduated to Phase II and a larger number of patients, ideally paired for age, sex, disease, pregnancy or not, and similar criteria. It would be given to four species in massive doses by various routes to determine its acute toxicity and to two species (rodent and non-rodent, usually rat and dog) for two to four weeks to indicate sub-acute toxicity and its effect on certain enzyme systems, other body chemistry and blood composition.

Phase II, by procedures difficult to understand, might show whether the drug will impair the female's ability to reproduce or, if she be pregnant, will abort her or cause her to bear a deformed or mutilated baby. As Giambalvo put it, "In the early stages of human studies, teratology and reproduction studies may be temporarily postponed by using only institutionalized female patients and/or women with not a ghost of a chance of becoming pregnant."

Then comes Phase III, the final test—one which hopefully will show whether the drug really helps the patient. Efficacy, it is called.

Phase III calls for the elimination of patients who respond to sugar pills and other placebos, for double blind studies in which neither patient nor doctor knows who gets the drug and who the placebo, for the elimination of the physician's bias (enthusiasm or dislike for particular drugs); it requires consideration of concomitant therapies and the grading of pain.

If aspirin survives Phase III and the New Drug Application stage, it goes on the market—but only under the watchful eyes of the Office of Drug Surveillance, which reviews adverse reactions and the effects of supplements, and the Office of Medical Review, which monitors medical advertising, medical devices, and over-the-counter drugs and helps out on the FDA's legal problems.

Actually, its acceptability would be doubtful, because aspirin has produced large liver tumors in rats, appeared to deplete human blood and tissue levels of vitamin C, and it had induced hemorrhage and other untoward side effects in adults with peptic ulcers. Some report that it exerts a "rebound effect" of clotting, with implied risks of strokes and heart attacks. Aspirin kills more than 100 Americans, mostly inquisitive children, each year.

Under literal application of the law, any doctor who tells a patient, "Take a couple of aspirin, and if you don't feel better in the morning, call me," risks a malpractice action.

Despite the law, aspirin is freely dispensed over the counter to anyone who can pay for it.

In some respects, Edward E. Rosenbaum, M.D., was the antithesis of Jacob. Now in private practice, Rosenbaum had been Clinical Professor of Medicine and founder of the Department of Rheumatology at the University of Oregon Medical School, a one-time intern in metabolic diseases at Michael Reese Hospital in Chicago, and, before and after his World War II service in the Army Medical Corps, a Fellow in Medicine at the Mayo Clinic. Rosenbaum was a broadly experienced, busy and prosperous physician.

Stocky, balding, middle-aged, Rosenbaum had a reputation in Portland as a hard-headed, feet-on-the-ground, show-me kind of doctor. He took nothing for granted, including patients' guesses and other doctors' diagnoses.

His home was luxurious and tasteful. He had a loving wife; and their four sons held the parents in high respect and affection. He had the rare—possibly unique—distinction of having three sons students at Harvard concurrently.

Rosenbaum had tested several new drugs for pharmaceutical houses and through his exacting requirements for evidence of safety and efficacy, had earned a reputation as being endowed with that precious scientific commodity, skepticism. It was this more than any other quality that made Stanley Jacob want to meet him and, if it proved feasible, work with him.

Jacob called Rosenbaum one October morning in 1963 and asked if he'd stop at his laboratory; he had a problem to talk over.

"I had a busy afternoon scheduled," Rosenbaum said. "I never will know why I canceled all appointments."

Rosenbaum had met Jacob only once or twice, and casually—Jacob had transplanted goat glands into one of his hypoparathyroid patients. Rosenbaum had heard rumors about DMSO, but he paid no attention to such patent fantasy.

Now Rosenbaum sat in a hard, straight-backed chair amid the swirl of laboratory smells and fixed Jacob with a shrewd clinical eye. He was wondering how the honored surgeon and scientist came by his glittering reputation.

Jacob held up a bottle of fluid. "You dab a little of this DMSO on the skin overlying the trouble," Jacob was saying, "and often within minutes the trouble vanishes. The headache disappears; sinuses clear; bruised tissues lose their ugly appearance; soreness leaves joints; pinkeye improves; bursitis subsides; many arthritics are helped.

"In less than one year of experiments, we've established multiple pharmacologic activities of DMSO." Jacob ticked them off on his fingers: "Analgesia, anti-inflammation, bacteriostasis, diuresis, tranquilizer, membrane penetration, transport and enhancement of other drugs, collagen solvent, non-specific immunity stimulant, and vasodilation."

When Rosenbaum gave no response, Jacob asked, "What do you think?"

"I think," Rosenbaum could have said, "that if you were my patient, I'd order you away for a long rest." Instead, he went to the door and closed it, and exhorted Jacob, "Look, Stan, you are secure now. You've got a good job. You've got prestige. Nothing's going to happen to you. But you're rocking the boat. Why don't you forget DMSO? Otherwise, you might destroy yourself and wind up without a job." Jacob's unhesitating response was, "Nothing doing."

This was the beginning of an all-weather research association.

Rosenbaum's initial experiences with DMSO were far from reassuring. His wife had a pain at the base of the thumb; DMSO didn't help. He tried it on a couple of other minor conditions. It was no good. Jacob had speculated that it might dissolve insulin and transport it through the skin, thus ending the need for insulin injections for diabetics. Rosenbaum promptly added insulin to DMSO and applied the product to his and Jacob's arms; it did not affect their blood sugar.

Jacob called Rosenbaum three or four or six times a day to inquire, "Have you used the DMSO? Have you seen anything yet?" On one occasion, Rosenbaum said, "Stanley, I have three arthritis patients in the office. They're willing to try DMSO. I'll keep them here for you." Jacob rushed down to Rosenbaum's office and applied the DMSO to the knees of the elderly women.

Within minutes of treatment, each of the patients professed to being free of pain—miraculously.

Jacob glowed.

Rosenbaum glowered. "I don't believe it," he said.

The next day Rosenbaum called the patients, and each confessed that she had not been helped at all. Furthermore, the DMSO had not given them a single moment's release from pain. Why had they lied? Each said approximately the same thing: "He was such a wonderful, earnest young doctor. I did not want to hurt his feelings."

Cynic, skeptic, doubter—whatever else Rosenbaum was, he was also tolerant and tenacious. He was convinced of one thing: DMSO did penetrate the skin—he had smelled it on his patients' breath. He also felt that Jacob was highly intelligent and utterly honest.

The two men met daily at lunch and talked DMSO. Jacob continued to call frequently to ask, "Ed, have you seen anything yet?"

A month or so after their first meeting, Rosenbaum said, "Look, Stan, I have yet to see one hopeful sign. Let's try it once more—in the rheumatology clinic at the medical school."

This was the clinic Rosenbaum had founded eleven years earlier and had headed up until he went into private practice three or four years ago. They went to the clinic that afternoon, selected a woman patient, explained the proposition and obtained her ready consent to the experiment. They gave the patient a small bottle of DMSO and instructed her in its use.

It occurred to the two physicians that, as a matter of courtesy, they should advise the chief of the clinic—Rosenbaum's successor—of their program.

And at this point Rosenbaum entered the gates of the hell in which Jacob had resided since shortly after tasting and testing DMSO.

"The chief of the clinic was very angry," Rosenbaum later told me. "He said DMSO was worthless in any rheumatic disease—our trials would bring disgrace upon his clinic—he would not permit us to use it."

They were made unwelcome at the clinic Rosenbaum had built.

When things looked blackest to Rosenbaum, he felt impelled to call Dean Baird and suggest that he reprimand Jacob—to save Baird from further embarrassment and Jacob from utter disgrace.

It was the first time Rosenbaum had ever called the dean.

"There's quite a stir at the school about DMSO," Rosenbaum finally blurted.

"Nobody believes Jacob," said the dean. "What do you think?"

Until this day, Rosenbaum doesn't know why he changed his course at that moment. Instead of warning Baird about Jacob, he heard himself saying, "I admire you for permitting him to go on with what appear to be negative results."

The dean laughed and hung up. Not many were tolerant of Jacob on the medical school campus.

On December 24, Christmas Eve, 1963, as Rosenbaum was closing his otherwise deserted office, a patient walked in with bursitis so painful that he could not move his shoulder. He had been unable to sleep the night before. Rosenbaum had him strip, examined him, and x-rayed his shoulder. He told the patient he had a new drug of unknown toxicity which might help. The patient begged him to try it.

Rosenbaum painted a small amount of DMSO on the man's shoulder and sat down and talked to him. He watched with some concern as the painted skin became red and itchy; and he could smell the oyster odor on the patient's skin and breath.

"After fifteen or twenty minutes, the patient looked at me and started to laugh," Rosenbaum told me. "He said, 'I can't believe it; the pain is gone.' I couldn't believe it either. I told him it probably was mere coincidence. I gave him a prescription for codeine and told him that if he had trouble, be sure and call me. He called me the next morning—Christmas Day. He told me he was almost free of pain.

"During the next two months, four more patients came to me with acute bursitis. Each was cured—I detest the word, but it almost applies—miraculously."

It was Rosenbaum's turn to do some telephoning. He caught Jacob just as he was leaving for a meeting in Florida. "Go in peace," Rosenbaum said. "Even I believe you have something."

Rosenbaum called Dr. Norman David, Head of the Department of Pharmacology, and at David's suggestion called the dean that evening at home. "I thought I heard a great sigh of relief, when I told him that DMSO was beginning to look good."

Ed Rosenbaum had earned his skepticism the hard way—by finding serious faults in the lessons learned at medical school, by discovering that the dogma and adages of his profession could be dreadfully wrong on occasion, that believing the clichés could lead to disaster, that the procedures and preparations considered safe and conservative in one edition of the medical manuals might be found dangerous and deadly in the next.

In 1952, Rosenbaum had the impression that chloroquine, the antimalarial, had helped his rheumatic patients. "Never trust clinical impressions," he reminded himself. For two years he and his associates conducted meticulous double-blind tests, and the data supported his observation handsomely. The facts and figures were pulled together in a carefully worded article and sent off to a journal. Before it was published, several other investigators were in print with sketchy data but the same conclusions. Credit to Rosenbaum et al., went down the drain.

Rosenbaum trusts no drug. Nor does he find implications in animal experiments very persuasive. Salvarsan and digitalis, he points out, are eminently safe in some laboratory animals in doses that would be a multiple of the lethal dose for humans; and Chloromycetin, which passed all lab tests and appeared safe in humans, was found to kill one in 68,000—a very lethal rate if you happen to be that susceptible person.

"It is often terribly hard to detect toxicity," Rosenbaum once told me. "A common assumption that if animals can survive a strong dose of Drug X, humans can take a small one, can be fatal reasoning.

"From the moment of conception, we face one near disaster after another. We face risks during residence in the womb, during our passage through the birth canal, walking across the street, or riding to the moon. In using drugs we must weigh the potential risks against the possible advantages. It makes a difference whether we are seeking relief of a minor pain or treating cancer."

DMSO in short order shattered a few more of Rosenbaum's idols.

A pharmacist friend had bothersome bursitis. Rosenbaum gave him a bottle of DMSO and told him to use it. The next morning the patient's wife called and said that for a while she had thought her husband had died—he had slept fourteen hours without stirring. It was his first sleep in many nights. The pharmacist, however, said he wasn't at all sure that DMSO deserved credit for the improvement.

One of the severest critics of Rosenbaum and Jacob borrowed DMSO and applied it to the bursitic shoulder of his policeman patient who was beyond other help. Within a half-hour the patient was almost pain-free. "What do you think happened?" Rosenbaum asked.

"There's no doubt about it," his critic said. "This case quite obviously has been misdiagnosed; whatever the condition, there has been a spontaneous remission." That point having been resolved, the physician asked earnestly: "Do you think I should buy Crown Zellerbach stock?"

An important professor came into Rosenbaum's office with a fresh bursitis of the shoulder. He said, "When I had an attack four years ago, the pain didn't respond even to morphine. The pain is back. I couldn't sleep last night, although I took large doses of codeine. I'm telling you now I don't believe what you and your fellow enthusiasts say about DMSO. But go ahead and try it on my shoulder anyway. I have nothing to lose." Terrified by the challenge of testing DMSO on so eminent and hostile a patient, Rosenbaum painted the shoulder with DMSO.

"He got the itch, the rash, the taste in his mouth," Rosenbaum recalled. "But while he was in my office, he couldn't be sure that he received any relief from pain." Rosenbaum gave him DMSO, told him to apply it every four hours if he could stand it, and sent him home. "He came back the next morning laughing. He told me it had worked."

Rosenbaum learned that patients, like drugs, should not be taken for granted.

Jacob faced the dilemma that confronts every scientist who has made a major discovery: When is the right time to claim credit? Unseemly haste could incite professional contempt. Delay could result in the glory going to a plagiarist.

There is a good deal of truth to the sardonic slogan: Publish or perish! Unless one gets something—almost anything—in the journals with reasonable regularity, he stands to lose face among his immediate superiors and associates, prestige in his field, and support from the granting agencies.

Scientific and medical journals do not pay their contributors for articles. On the contrary, authors pay for reprints. And considering the quality of the articles, this is as it should be 90 per cent of the time.

For their services, most editors earn only whatever honors accrue from having their names on the masthead. And this too is as it should be; it makes clear where the blame belongs.

Scientists, doctors and—let us not forget, engineers and educators—have managed to construct awkward, pompous jargons which not only are unintelligible to the unwashed public but sometimes beyond the understanding of the inventors as well, a confounding curse of tongues, a cryptographic code lacking a key. The archaic, anti-semantic prose, the pretentious Greco-Latin hybrid terms, the obfuscatory, pseudo-modest passive voice, the tedious and meaningless technical detail, the open bridges in logic, the anachronisms, the ambiguities and obscurantism in data, the craven "it is tempting to conclude" sort of non-conclusion, and the timid "may warrant further investigation" cop-out—all these contribute to the illiteracy of the professions. One survey showed that the average doctor reads fewer than three journals a month. Scientists glance through more publications than that, and some of the articles, they may actually read. By and large, however, the 15–25,000 or so medical and scientific journals represent a modern monument to the Tower of Babel.

Journals sometimes refuse to publish articles because the material is too new or too explosively significant. Many of the great scientists have found it difficult or impossible to find an outlet for some of their most challenging papers. The young and relatively unknown, especially, have been denied credit, in this wise, for work that others repeated and reported and sometimes won awards for years later.

Besides their journals, scientists have one other medium of communication—the professional meeting. This event comes in many sizes. There are small get-togethers of between ten and a hundred scientists or physicians who gather in an isolated but comfortable resort to mull over a medical or scientific problem for several days. Usually, the speakers know each other well; they have spoken and listened to one another for years; sometimes any one of them can recite, without notes or prompting, what any or all of the others can be expected to say.

There are large conventions where one or two or three thousand papers will be droned out before numerous scattered audiences of mostly bored people who don't hear, or understand, or care what is said and who are too beaten to protest against the illegible tables and the meaningless charts and graphs shown on the screen.

The most mature and candid will confess that the meetings

33

have come to depress them, that they are an ill-afforded drain on time better spent in their laboratories.

There are exceptions to the foregoing. A few scientists and physicians do a creditable job of educating others. Their papers are clear, erudite, significant, stimulating. Their lectures awaken an audience and send them away with new ideas, new zest, new means and methods of exploring new areas. And, in some, a sense of outrage.

Gifted with total recall of facts that he considered solid and significant, remembering precisely where to look for data published by others, knowing exactly what he wanted to say and how to say it so that it could be understood easily, Jacob found neither lecturing nor writing a great chore. He could dictate in a couple of hours a first-rate paper for which some scientists would take a month or two off to write badly. Before he had heard of DMSO, he had published about forty papers in prestigious journals, most of which had attracted considerable attention. He was to become the author of medical books that sold widely.

Jacob's lectures were lucid, his critiques incisive. A one-time champion debater, he was a formidable foe where facts were at issue and he was skilled in taking specious arguments and fatuous orators apart.

Jacob had one great failing, however; he was unable to lie or dissemble or equivocate. Even to newsmen. For this weakness, which, as it turned out, was unpardonable in his profession, he was to pay dearly.

Portland is fortunate in having two highly competent medical and science writers—Marge Davenport of the *Oregon Journal,* a youthful mother of five youngsters, and Ann Sullivan, of the *Oregonian,* a mature, well-stacked brunette of the old aggressive school of journalism. Both writers heard the first rumors about DMSO; they checked then with Jacob, who told them the truth; and although they were keen competitors, they refrained from

34

breaking the story, because premature publication would embarrass Jacob before that large professional conglomerate known as his "peers." They were holding back a medical matter of high journalistic and public interest; but they did so long after Portland physicians had noised the news abroad and were buying Crown Zellerbach stock.

Jacob's housekeeper told the reporters that after she had had her swollen and painful jaw painted with DMSO, following extraction of several teeth, symptoms of an old stroke improved; her uncertain gait became steady; she could take a pen in her paralyzed hand and write.

Agricultural researchers along the Hood River had shown Miss Sullivan apple trees which had been withered and old; a shot of DMSO into the growing, juicy cambial layer, just under the bark, made them suddenly lush with leaves and with other signs of youth.

Miss Sullivan's octogenarian baby-sitter fell and injured her thumb and wrist. Ann told me, "We put some DMSO on that big, green, pulsating hand, and, as we watched, the swelling and pain left." She said the UCLA football team used DMSO liberally —"They won the conference championship, and some of the team lost their girls because of the DMSO odor."

"Stanley is a generous man who lives only for others," Miss Sullivan said. "He has not the slightest desire for money.

"He is the complete genius. He can turn off all his personal troubles and give himself completely to what he feels must be done for others. In this case, DMSO had to be made available to sick and suffering people. His motive is that simple.

"He likes women. He is adored by the nurses. It is possible that his appeal to women may account in part for the bitterness of his male critics. It could be biological.

"He is hard-driving and unhappy. He has no hobbies, no sports. He has no time to play. At parties, he'll toy with a drink for a while and then take off. When he comes to dinner, he eats, sits on the davenport, falls asleep, gets up and goes home—or, more often, back to the lab.

"He doesn't spend money on himself. He has no possessions. He doesn't care about cars, or clothes, but he wears his clothes well and he is handsome. He doesn't dislike anyone. And he just can't understand why anyone would dislike him."

The day came when Marge Davenport and Ann Sullivan had to release the story. By all the practices of good journalism, by whatever code might be involved, by all the tenets of human communication, common decency and common sense, they had to print the facts. They explained this to Jacob; and, while he would have liked to appease his critics by holding off until the facts were published in a scientific journal, he realized that the choice was not his or the reporters'.

The precipitating circumstance was the filing of a contract in Salem, the state capital. In this public document, which was available not only to the press but to any man, woman or child who cared to see it, Crown Zellerbach and the state of Oregon, through its Board of Higher Education, became partners in the patented medical uses of DMSO. The patents actually were requested for Herschler and Jacob as representing their respective institutions. The formal document described the major uses to which DMSO had been put, and the information became public property from that moment.

Portland newspapers carried the story on page one on December 10, 1963. But for all the excitement it stirred outside Oregon, it could have been buried "back among the truss ads," as they say. The wire services brushed it off with a perfunctory couple of paragraphs, which many papers ignored completely. The *Oregonian* later carried an editorial bewailing the effete Eastern attitude toward earthshaking news originating in Indian Country.

Then, on Wednesday, December 18, the New York *Times* gave the story its seal of approval. It played on page one Robert K.

Plumb's piece about DMSO's "creating a stir in medical circles in Portland." That was all that was needed.

Crown Zellerbach stock jumped $5.50 a share that day to $60.25. *Newsweek's* medical editor, Matt Clark, contributed a lucid account in the issue of December 23. *U. S. News & World Report* followed on December 30 with an article on the testing of "a drug that could open up a new era in medicine." *Life* and *Saturday Evening Post* writers began looking into the story for future spectaculars.

Then, for almost two years, articles were frequent in almost all major publications in the United States and in many abroad.

None of the principals—Jacob, Rosenbaum, the university, and, certainly, neither Herschler nor Crown Zellerbach—was happy about the publicity. (Crown stock quotations had fallen back to normal when the corporation pointed out that DMSO could not amount to more than a drop in its corporate bucket). Everyone involved wished that the press could and would have held off until the DMSO story could be obtained from medical and scientific journals.

To set the record straight, it must be said that:

1) The first written accounts of DMSO as a drug were submitted to medical journals between four and six months before the news broke in the public press; and

2) The first oral description was delivered to scientific audiences more than two months prior to the news break.

In all instances, nobody in authority believed that a compound with DMSO's versatile biological activity could possibly exist. The situation was not new. Doubt of this sort had delayed major scientific effort since before Galileo.

During the summer of 1963, Jacob and Herschler had written a paper on the basic pharmacology of DMSO and sent it, in turn, to *Science, Nature* and *Surgery*. All of them said no, thanks. Obviously, they regarded as preposterous the claim that the authors had discovered seven primary biological actions in one very simple solvent.

In October 1963, Jacob presented his report before the Surgical Biology Club, which meets each year just prior to the annual meeting of the American College of Surgeons. The members listened to his lecture with interest—and amusement. Many thought he was ribbing them; and they shook their heads and chuckled at this rare brand of humor. He offered to report to the Society of University Surgeons; they turned him down.

In effect, the efforts to publish eventually became a hectic, last-ditch search for cover. Patents for DMSO medical uses had been applied for and the partnership papers, joining the Oregon Board of Higher Education and Crown Zellerbach, had been drawn up and had to become public before the year's end. In the race against time, Jacob, along with his friends and associates, had run a poor second.

Jacob and all who were associated with him breathed a little more easily when it looked as though DMSO would qualify for "respectability." Arrangements finally were made for oral presentation before "peers" and also for the drug's debut in formal medical and scientific literature.

Jacob reported on the pharmacology of DMSO before the faculty of the University of Oregon Medical School. There never had been so unruly a session in the history of the institution. The auditorium was hot with the heat of more than 100 keyed-up faculty members. Plus a few research assistants and students, all of them solidly in the seats, aisles and all open spaces. The questions were leading and pointed, like switchblades. Tempers flared. Some were heard to cry out, "Liar!" "Quack!" "Charlatan!" It was Jacob's first intellectual mugging.

A day or so later, Dunphy, the Chief of Surgery, summoned Jacob into his office and told him that a few faculty members had asked Dean Baird to fire Jacob. Dunphy was upset and embarrassed; but inasmuch as he was about to leave for a job at the University of California Medical School in San Francisco, he did not pursue the point. The friendship, which dated back to Jacob's residency at Harvard, survived.

Jacob, Margaret Bischel (a senior medical student) and Herschler submitted an article on "DMSO: A New Concept in Pharmacotherapy" to *Current Therapeutic Research*, a journal of limited circulation. The article appeared early in 1964 over an editorial apology: "The above serves to record a most unusual series of biological responses to a widely known compound which has not been previously used as a medicinal agent. The authors give assurance that several colleagues are currently assembling the data on their clinical observations for publication at an early date." It was only because Dr. Norman David, a sympathetic associate editor, had intervened, that the piece ever saw the light of day.

Another article, by Jacob and Rosenbaum, on the first seven patients treated for bursitis, was submitted in January and appeared in *Northwest Medicine* in March 1964, and still another on DMSO and arthritis in the April issue. *Northwest Medicine*, a readable and informative journal, has as its editor Herbert L. Hartley, M.D., who likes to have solid reasons for accepting an article and equally valid grounds for rejecting one. He knows most of his contributors personally—those he publishes and those he rejects—and it is very hard to find a literate and reasonable doctor in the Pacific Northwest who doesn't swear by Herb Hartley and *Northwest Medicine*.

The legitimization of DMSO—if articles in two professional journals could be called that—was a mixed bag. It opened the floodgates of powerful prose for the news media. Instead of appeasing the critics, professional publication seemed to embitter them more; one young Ph.D. dropped into Jacob's lab one morning only long enough to say, "I have come all the way from the state of Florida to see the author of the most preposterous paper which has ever appeared in the medical literature."

Professional publication set off a scramble among doctors everywhere for some of this precious stuff, DMSO, and while many of them used it with common sense and caution, others initiated an epidemic of wild, senseless, irrational experimentation on humans. Some experimentalists lacked the scientific background to treat white mice.

Dr. H. P. Dygert, a part-time faculty member, could have spoken for most, if not all, the dissident elements at the medical school in deploring "the unforgivably unscientific manner in which the investigation has been carried out or the publicity offered." In a letter to the editor of *Northwest Medicine,* he said, "The inherent dangers in this situation, both legal and in the potential harm to medicine's position of leadership in health matters in this country, should our position be challenged, is uncalculable." He ended his reprimand with a cryptic observation in classical medical journalese: "I urge all persons in a position to influence this situation, and particularly the University of Oregon School of Medicine, to review this entire matter and to attempt as rapidly as possible to bring it into proper perspective."

Dygert protested that one of his patients with obstructive emphysema and ulcerative colitis had asked for DMSO treatment and had been accepted "until I intervened."

DMSO, an investigative drug, was distributed in 1964 under the name Dymasol. Zirin Corporation, in offering it for "fantastic relief, almost instantly, from most of the time and money-losing aches and pains of horses," quoted liberally from newspapers and magazines and acclaimed DMSO as "one of the most important medical events of the century—comparable to the discoveries of penicillin, insulin, and the life-saving vaccines."

"This epoch-making drug is unique in so many ways that it would require a substantial volume to detail them—it is probably the first drug administered to more human beings than to animals for clinical investigation," the ad said.

Those who knew DMSO best might have agreed with all or a good deal of the advertising. But they winced, nevertheless. The hard sell pitch did not help the cause of DMSO. Or of Jacob, who was being battered by other problems, and who was relieved when Dymasol was withdrawn.

41

Some faculty members who formerly smiled greetings now would nod curtly or look away as they passed Jacob in the hallways. Itinerant colleagues were damning his findings as having no validity.

Whereas, until DMSO, Jacob had been elected to learned societies and professional organizations with unanimous and enthusiastic endorsement, he now ceased getting invitations to join. Twice he had been proposed for membership in the Pacific Coast Surgical Society, and twice, after bitter fighting, under charges of quackery and charlatanism, he was rejected. At the third meeting, he was accepted; his champions—Dr. Clare Peterson and Dr. William Krippaehne, surgeon friends and associates at the medical school—launched a counterattack which made a narrow majority of the members vote him in.

Jacob's opposition here came exclusively from downtown surgeons, many of them with quite ordinary academic credentials. (Jacob had and has no enemies in his own department of surgery.)

By way of contrast, Jacob had been given the largest number of votes of any candidate the year he was elected to the Society of University Surgeons, strictly major league; but that was in 1962, before anyone knew of his interest in DMSO.

Jacob was elected also to the Surgical Biology Club, an elite group of fellows of the American College of Surgeons; he was one of only two or three who were not departmental chairmen. This appointment took place in 1960—two years before DMSO—and was on the basis of his status not so much as a surgeon but as a scientist.

About the only other group Jacob wanted to join for reasons of professional prestige was the American Surgical Association. He gave up hope when he learned of the bitterness of the Pacific Coast Surgical Society members.

He soon noticed coolness even among some old acquaintances at the meetings of the American College of Surgeons, in which he had been enrolled in 1960. The ACS is large, authoritative, progressive and responsible. As in all professional societies, there is an element of politics in the election of its leaders, and, consequently, the quality of its service varies somewhat from one administration to the next; but, by and large, the college tries to fulfill its obligations to the public as well as to its members.

At this time, with a few faculty members imploring Dean Baird to get rid of Jacob "for the good of the school," Jacob sent a report on DMSO to Dunphy, his friend and immediate superior. He had treated some patients with precarious conditions—he listed a score of them—and, seemingly, with good or excellent response. Dunphy sent Jacob a note saying, "This smacks of Andrew Ivy." (Dr. Ivy was the prominent educator at the University of Illinois Medical School who was then supporting Krebiozen, a controversial cancer drug.)

"Dr. Dunphy didn't want to hurt me," Jacob explained. "I think he was trying to save me. He was the one who arranged for me to write my book *Structure and Function in Man*.

"At about this time, Dr. Dunphy said at one luncheon meeting —and I'll never forget it, because it was so unusual—that he had had a dream that the DMSO matter had been turned over to the National Academy of Sciences."

Inasmuch as that was more than eight years before the National Academy did agree to look into the DMSO matter, Dunphy's experience may have been more a vision than a dream.

Until DMSO, Stanley Jacob was buttonholed regularly at large medical meetings to accept positions elsewhere. There was the chance to work with the pioneering cardiovascular man, Dr. Adrian Kantrowitz, then at Downstate Medical Center in Brooklyn; he could have become Professor of Surgery at Temple and Chairman of the Department of Surgery at Albert Einstein Medical Center in Philadelphia. He could have gone to Louisiana State University as an associate professor and worked with those who devised regional perfusion and other imaginative and highly successful techniques in cancer surgery.

Jacob liked Portland, its medical school, Baird, Peterson, Krippaehne, the faculty and students; he listened politely to the offers—and said without hesitation, "Thanks, but no." That was between 1959 and 1963. For the next decade, he was not approached to take work elsewhere.

Periodically, research advisory committees meet to study scientists' applications—like Jacob's—for grants, to discuss them, and to render a grade and an opinion on each of them for the benefit of the governmental or voluntary agency being solicited for support. The committees or councils are composed of panels, each of a dozen or so reputable scientists who consider projects within or akin to their specialty. The committee members serve as a favor to science generally and to the agency, and they receive only their out-of-pocket expenses for their day or two in New York or Washington. A fringe benefit quite often is that the panel members themselves have grant applications to be debated by the committee (they absent themselves for a few minutes during this discussion); and they are in a position to say a good word for a friend or a sour one for an enemy.

Some feel that a scientist could be a rapist, a drunk, a child molester, or a devotee of plain and fancy perversion and still receive his grant if he avoids professional flamboyance. This is most adroitly done by publishing a great many wordy and highly technical papers about insignificant work. Whenever a project reaches

44

the point where it is about to produce a cure for a serious disease, however, the grant is in jeopardy; it may not be renewed. The most sophisticated practitioners of grantsmanship do not publish or advise committees of an earthshaking development in their studies until later, when they have under way a new project of a more or less bland, amorphous nature.

Advisory committee members, or the granting agency's employees, draw upon a strange lexicon to damn a scientist or a project that is not to their liking. "He is very enthusiastic about this," is a surefire way of condemning an application. Or, "Oh, yes, I read articles in the newspapers about this work." Or, "Good man, Jones, brimming over with new ideas. Very imaginative fellow."

Stanley Jacob had worked on a lot of grants from an assortment of government and other agencies. He had no trouble getting grants, despite the fact that he was honest, unable to dissemble, and, you should excuse the expression, enthusiastic. None of his studies posed any immediate threat to the solid structure of conventional medicine. There were implications but not immediate applications in nerve resection for peptic ulcer, hormones for hemorrhagic shock and kidney transplants, enzyme activity in pancreatitis and in various surgical emergencies, the removal of lobes of the liver, bone marrow transplants to overcome lethal x-rays, the supercooling of hearts and other organs for transplantation, the effect of body cooling (in surgery) on the brain, and stomach freezing for ulcers. None of these studies yet had reached the stage where doctors were confronted with the prospect of having to learn new practices in medicine; that came later.

Then came DMSO. Grants that Jacob had obtained without effort became hard to get.

The year 1964 had its sweet as well as sour seasons.

Jacob made extraordinary progress in extending his clinical trials with DMSO to such challenging areas as nerve blindness, baldness, various infections, gangrene from several causes, disc troubles, injuries of all sorts, dystrophies, paraplegia, mental diseases, diseases of the digestive tract from glossitis to hemorrhoiditis, from psoriasis of the scalp to athlete's foot, and disturbances stemming from all the external and internal organs.

Jacob began his clinical experiments gingerly; but as animal work indicated the basic biological safety of DMSO and his clinical observations showed it to be a drug probably without parallel for both safety and efficacy in an amazing number of conditions, he became emboldened. He tested the solvent's mysterious powers against fearsome ailments considered difficult or impossible to treat effectively.

At this time the officials of the Food and Drug Administration were encouraging and co-operative. On March 18, 1964, FDA, Crown and University of Oregon representatives met in Room 2029 of the FDA Building back East. Present for the FDA were Drs. Frances O. Kelsey, G. W. Schepers (pathologist), E. I. Goldenthal (pharmacologist), and J. A. Kaiser (also pharmacology); for Crown, Dr. W. M. Hearon, two lawyers, Vincent Kleinfeld and Richard Nelson, and Bob Herschler; for the medical school, Drs. Jacob and Norman David.

"The FDA representatives seemed anxious to do everything possible to permit further testing of DMSO," Jacob told me later. "They pointed out that DMSO was a very versatile drug; and because of this they were a little apprehensive as to how many IND applications might be filed to test not only DMSO alone but DMSO in combinations with various other pharmacologically active substances.

"Dr. Kelsey said the number of combinations could be a hundred or more, representing a formidable challenge for a bureau that already was overburdened."

David produced more than 100 pages of toxicological data on DMSO which had been compiled by medical school investigators; and Jacob reviewed his methods of application, dosages and results, most of them necessarily of a preliminary nature.

Jacob described clinical trials at Oregon State Hospital in which mental patients were being given about a teaspoonful of DMSO orally every day. Although members of the staff had themselves taken this dosage for some time and had administered DMSO orally in large doses to animals without serious reaction, the FDA officials said these experiments must cease because there was not sufficient animal data to warrant them.

"Dr. Kelsey and her group seemed almost apologetic," Jacob said, "and they expressed the hope that the work would be continued since the goals obviously were worthwhile. Dr. Schepers said we could start our clinical testing again at Oregon State Hospital as soon as we had one month's toxicity data. He suggested running a series of dogs on a one-administration-a-day basis for only one month, autopsying a dog each month, and, if no abnormalities occurred, obtaining a permit from the FDA to start again the study at the hospital."

At this point, the FDA could not have been more reasonable. And, consequently or coincidentally, science and medicine in the United States were in a fairly healthy shape.

Even during this period of peace, however, the FDA was responding to pressures from politicians in Congress and ambitious officers within its own structure. Publicity and power were to be had in assuring the public that thalidomide-type disasters would not happen here. They were right. But another kind of calamity could have been building up as an overreaction to a danger which had passed.

The drug houses became skeptical, then curious about DMSO and, finally, interested. There were mixed feelings; DMSO had to be an inexpensive product and, if it lived up to its early promise, it could substitute for a large number of pharmaceuticals which had cost the drug houses vast sums to develop and now were costing the public a lot of money to consume.

It fell to Ed Rosenbaum to handle the greater part of transactions. He had tested several new preparations for pharmaceutical companies; he knew their officers and clinical advisors; he knew their psychology, their habits, their language. And under Rosenbaum's guidance, drug house enthusiasm for DMSO rose— and so did drug house investments in expensive laboratory and clinical testing. As the FDA's demands on DMSO became more stringent, the costs of testing rose to $10 million, then to $15 million and beyond. If and when DMSO is ever marketed, it may represent one of the industry's most investigated and invested-in drugs.

Rosenbaum told me later of episodes during those turbulent times.

Crown's executives invited him and Jacob to lunch occasionally. "I was impressed with their total ignorance in the field of drug evaluation," he said. "They seemed to think they were dealing with an ordinary chemical compound and it could be handled as any other pulp or paper product.

"They were fine, pleasant men; but like all corporation executives, they exhibited a great drive for profits. When things were going well, we were the greatest people in the world. Crown always gave us a free lunch and occasionally sent us a Christmas card."

Rosenbaum applauded the care with which Crown selected drug houses to conduct clinical investigations. "They were determined to pick the most ethical and reliable drug firms," he said.

Rosenbaum reported that after being courted by Geigy, he recommended them for a license, but Geigy later became disenchanted with DMSO.

Ed called DMSO to the attention of Max Tishler, a dynamic figure in the pharmaceutical industry, president of the Merck Institute and director of medical research. Merck assigned Dr. Richard Brobyn—young, sharp and knowledgeable enough to entertain enthusiasms—to investigate. Brobyn dug, felt that he had struck pay dirt, and reported accordingly.

Rosenbaum said Squibb was among the first to confirm the fact that DMSO would transport some drugs across tissue membranes. He didn't have much information about the role played by American Home Products.

Syntex showed considerable enthusiasm, for a while at least. They assigned Dr. Gerhard Boost, a former thoracic surgeon then in Salem, Oregon, and a man with a high sense of ethics, to undertake extensive clinical studies. It was Boost's feeling that any information which might preserve human life could not become a secret to be held in commercial trust indefinitely.

The American Schering Corporation undertook clinical studies under the direction of an able pediatrician, Dr. Sam Bukantz of St. Louis. The studies apparently ended abortively when Bukantz transferred to Hoffmann-La Roche Corporation.

Jacob, meanwhile, had to cope not only with the angry men in his audiences, the bitter critics on his campus and the journal editors but also with the massive, impersonal, immutable structure of medicine. Most of the disciples he won were unwilling to face the cold resistance, if not abuse, which impeded his own progress.

49

One of the dedicated devotees was Dr. Morris Green.

Green was among those who lingered after Stanley Jacob's 1964 Boston lecture and the question-and-answer period that followed. He was obviously excited. Normally a quiet man, he elbowed his way to the front of the small circle surrounding Jacob in the auditorium of Beth Israel Hospital and began firing questions, mainly queries on the chemistry and biochemistry of DMSO. After all the others had disappeared into the warmth of this May evening, Green continued to pose questions.

Morris Nathan Green, Ph.D., could be described as a sort of medium-man—medium height, medium build, medium bald, medium gray hair, at almost fifty-four years, medium middle age, and about midway on the ladder to success in science.

Green's background in academia was broad and rich—B.S. from M.I.T.; A.M. and University Fellow in Medical Sciences at Boston University; M.S. (Biological Chemistry) University of Michigan; and, when he was thirty-four years old and after ten years in various research and teaching posts at several universities, his Ph.D. (Bacteriology) from the University of Pennsylvania. He had had additional post-doctoral research and teaching jobs at Iowa State, Pennsylvania and the University of Missouri before he went to Harvard Medical School at age forty-one, first as a Research Associate in Surgery, Associate in Surgical Research (at Beth Israel Hospital) and finally, in 1955, Research Associate in (Clinical) Pathology, the Children's Hospital and the Children's Cancer Research Foundation, and Research Associate in Pathology, Harvard Medical School. Green was very active in the Jewish community's educational affairs. He belonged to five learned societies.

If Green's star was not the brightest in the glittering galaxy he inhabited, he at least thoroughly relished the intellectual fare dished up by the resident and visiting geniuses. He came to Jacob's lecture, his curiosity roused by the news accounts he had read but without the deep prejudice that so often preceded the visiting surgeon. He told me about it later.

"After hearing the presentation," Green said, "I became excited. I had two thoughts: the first was that the DMSO principle was a natural for forcing anti-tumor agents into tumors and, therefore, might improve the results at lower dosages. The second was that DMSO should be good for depolymerizing, or breaking up, the mucus in cystic fibrosis."

At the meeting, he made the cystic fibrosis suggestion but kept the tumor implication for discussion with colleagues at Children's Cancer Research Foundation.

"I went home that night in a dither," Green said. "No doubt, many who listened to Jacob got the impression he was talking about Lydia Pinkham's Vegetable Compound. But in my mind, he had opened up a new scientific principle with wide application."

The very next day, Green was admitted to the office of Dr. Harry Schwachman at the Children's Cancer Research Foundation. He was ecstatic. Schwachman, an expert in cystic fibrosis, did not excite easily. But he listened politely as Green explained that DMSO might clear the breathing apparatus of the viscid blocks which often lead to death.

"He said, no, he didn't want to be the first to try it," Green said. "But as a result of my suggestion, the Schwachman group did modify the iontophoresis test to stimulate the production of sweat; the electrolytes are elevated in cystic fibrosis. They tried my suggestion that pilocarpine dissolved in DMSO be used to make babies produce enough sweat for diagnosis; and it worked."

Green said that he also sought out Dr. Thomas Hall to propose that he combine anti-cancer drugs with DMSO. Hall, head of chemotherapy, told Green to talk with Charlotte Maddock, M.D., who was in charge of the experimental tumor laboratory at Children's Cancer Research Foundation. To Dr. Maddock, Green suggested that a tumor be implanted into mice and that the site then be swabbed with the DMSO-anti-cancer drug combination. Maddock agreed.

As the months passed without word from Maddock, Green

concluded sadly that another good idea had gone down the drain. But he just couldn't get the idea of DMSO as an anti-cancer agent out of his system. He corresponded regularly with Jacob, hoping someone would test his theory.

Beset by hostilities at home and disdain elsewhere, Jacob, nonetheless, never lost his sense that DMSO someday would triumph. An endless succession of unexpected events dispelled any tendencies toward depression.

There was the time, for example, the Texas doctors had to play God. They had to decide whether to let the little black boy die decently and quickly or to risk heroic measures which might inflict disability or an ugly and painful death.

The boy, aged seven, had entered a hospital in great pain, his belly distended grotesquely with peritonitis. The surgeons opened him up, found the small intestine gangrenous and the large intestine twisted and completely blocked. They removed his digestive tract from just below the stomach to the mid-bowel. The operation didn't leave much intestinal surface through which ingested nutrients could pass into the bloodstream. And so—sick and slowly starving—he was moved to the pediatric services of Wilford Hall, Lackland Air Force Base Hospital, near San Antonio, Texas. It was just before the Yuletide; the spirit of the Magi may have prevailed. Death is not a fitting Christmas gift for a child.

Intravenous feeding of high caloric fluids and electrolytes failed to compensate for the diarrhea and malabsorption, nor did it stem

53

the wasting of muscle, the progressive weight loss, the anemia—the deterioration of what had been a little boy.

When it became almost impossible to find veins for injections, three of the Air Force doctors—Lt. Col. Robert E. Smith, Capt. Andrew M. Hegre, Jr., and Capt. Clement N. Rieffel, Jr.—decided to undertake an experiment that some would have considered a journey into fantasy; they would try to feed the dying boy through his skin.

The doctors mixed a glucose solution with an equal amount of 100 per cent DMSO and swabbed it on the boy's skin. Gradually the stuff dissipated, and at the end of twenty minutes, serum tests showed, it was gone completely—into the lad's system. Then they added to DMSO some vitamins, fats, proteins, minerals; and he was "fed" dermally five or six "meals" a day.

It was touch and go, but during the first thirteen days on this regimen the boy's weight rose from 32.75 pounds to a glorious thirty-five pounds; and during the next week he added still another 1.25 pounds. At this point, however, his anemia became acute, his weight dropped to thirty-four pounds, and it was necessary to cut through the flesh to find a vein capable of being catheterized for injections of vitamin B12, iron and other essentials. Once again, flesh began to fill out the bony outlines, and by July 5, he tipped the scales at a remarkable thirty-seven pounds. Then, on July, a slight but sudden rise in temperature indicated infection—possibly caused by the indwelling catheter—and on July 10 the catheter was removed.

The boy did well for the next few days. But on July 15 at 3 A.M., the hour when, some say, human resistance is at its lowest, his lungs became congested and his breathing labored. He went into a coma; and, despite desperate measures—including a feeding tube inserted into his jugular vein, antibiotics, transfusions, electrolytes, suctioning of his fluid-filled lungs, and other tactics—he quietly died on July 16. At 3 A.M.

The autopsy showed pneumonia the cause of death and "no evidence of toxicity from DMSO."

The doctors said their tests "left little doubt that the nutrients crossed through the skin barrier in usable form"; but they added that the replacement of fluids and electrolytes remained a problem. "Supplemental feeding through the skin with DMSO *does* seem possible," they concluded.

An increasing volume of encouraging mail also buoyed up Jacob's spirits. This is a sample:

Dear Stanley:

The patient is now doing fine. One of the strangest features in this case, Reiter's disease [a probably non-venereal syndrome resembling gonococcal arthritis], was the fact that he had failed to respond to carloads of antibiotics, steroids and everything else you can imagine. Following his splendid response, I discontinued DMSO with one-half of the bottle left. For the sake of experimentation, I put him back on small doses of prednisolone, and he continued to remain afebrile and practically free of joint symptoms.

The steroid was gradually reduced to zero, and he is doing perfectly well with aspirin. This is strange and bizarre, to say the least. He was, by any clinical standards, a critically ill man when I first began to administer the DMSO.

Like the thousands of others who have benefited from your observations, I shall always be grateful for coming to my aid when I was watching the poor guy suffer and wishing that he was dead.

X.Y.Z., M.D.

Dept. of Urology

X College of Medicine

Jacob and Rosenbaum were invited by Dr. Gerhard Laudahn, Director of Schering AG, the German drug house, to a special one-day symposium on DMSO in Berlin in July 1965. Both men gratefully and hopefully accepted; they were pretty well worn out by the battles at home and thought that, even if the trip amounted to another series of conflicts, at least it might be refreshing to fight on foreign ground.

Berlin turned out to be a joy. They were met at the airport by Laudahn and Dr. Heinz John of Berlin, and they were shown the city and taken to Laudahn's home. They were guests of honor at the session; and, socially, they were given red-carpet hospitality. Most gratifying of all was the intelligence and enthusiasm shown by the 150 German, Austrian, Scandinavian, Swiss and other European participants in the morning scientific and afternoon clinical sessions. Those who spoke did so from knowledge; those who asked questions were curious and courteous. None seemed disposed to argue for the sake of argument.

"The thing that impressed me," Rosenbaum said later, "was that while the Germans started their DMSO studies later than American pharmaceutical houses did, they seemed to be ahead of us."

Late in 1965, when things looked dark for DMSO, Dr. Charlotte Maddock walked into the laboratory of Dr. Morris Green at Children's Cancer Research Foundation in Boston.

"She was all excited," Green later told me. "She had started some experiments on the P-1534 tumor many months earlier—and all animals treated with a DMSO combination were surviving in good shape."

"P-1534" originally had been a spontaneous leukemia in mice. When it was implanted in muscle or under the skin, it grew locally, infiltrated promptly and killed the mouse in about fourteen days. When treated early, it responded pretty well to either of two drugs, 5-FU or actinomycin D. With DMSO/5-FU, some mice were not only cured but they also became immune to the tumor.

Green shared Maddock's excitement. Together they tested several other drug combinations against more experimental tumors, with and without DMSO. In almost all cases—there was an exception or two—the cure or the dramatic response depended on whether DMSO had been used in the combination. DMSO alone, however, was generally ineffective.

56

L-1210 leukemia, which kills the mouse in about eight days, takes twice as long to kill if a common anti-cancer drug, cytoxan, is used, but the preparation has to be shot into the belly cavity —intraperitoneally, as they say. The same result (15.3 days survival) was achieved with DMSO-cytoxan merely dabbed on the skin.

Significant results—generally on the order of doubling the survival of animals treated with DMSO plus any of such agents as 5-FU, CRI-3, cytoxan, thio-TEPA and 6-MP—were reported in such induced animal tumors as other leukemias, cancer of the connective tissue and bone, and melanoma, or "black cancer," of the pigment-producing cells of the skin.

A great deal of work had to be done to find effective drug combinations and establish dosages, proportions and routes of administration. In one or two instances, DMSO plus actinomycin D had shortened the animal's survival somewhat.

Green and Maddock sent to Dr. Sidney Farber, the famous director of Children's Cancer Research Foundation on December 3, 1965, an account of their experiences. They offered a summary of the complete disintegration wrought by DMSO/5-FU on experimental mouse cancers, and they said in closing:

Since the experimental work that you are being presented with, together with added material that reaffirms the fact the topical applications of a cytotoxic agent in DMSO, when properly applied as to dosage and schedule, may be successful in slowing down growth and even eradicating tumor, the following question arises. Is a preliminary publication in order with what material we shall shortly have, and if so, should it be readied for rapid publication in say "Science" or "Proc. Soc. Exper. Biol. and Med." or should we proceed at a more leisurely pace and aim for presenting this at the Association for Cancer Research meetings in May?

We would appreciate your wise guidance.

A couple of months later, Farber gave the paper his blessing. The approved draft came back from the front office with DMSO taken out of the title, and it was delivered by Maddock at the AACR annual meeting in Denver.

Green, after clearing it with Maddock, arranged to board a train in Denver for Portland, where, on Jacob's invitation, he would lecture the University of Oregon Medical School faculty.

For Green, Maddock and even DMSO things were going great.

As late as September 8, 1965, all seemed well. A freshet of facts from controlled studies was streaming into the computers of participating drug houses. More and more scientists were testing DMSO against plant pathology, mouse cancer, an array of diseases in laboratory animals, and a rapidly broadening range of conditions in man. Some biochemical rationales for DMSO's numerous biological activities were beginning to emerge; and, perhaps most important of all, DMSO was opening the inner and outer membranes of cells to expose life's great secrets that lay hidden behind them.

On September 8, Merck Sharp & Dohme Laboratories sent out to all investigators under their auspices an advisory memorandum on the emerging role of DMSO in experimental medicine. The prospects for the release of DMSO as a prescription drug looked very bright.

Here are some of the points made by Merck, as I have reduced them to capsule form:

INTRODUCTION

DMSO has been under investigation for over a year. This revised summary reflects the clinical experience of that time. It is intended as a guide for investigators in regard to indications for use, dosage, method of administration, etc., and it provides information concerning precautions and possible adverse reactions.

DMSO therapy is constantly changing. New indications are developing and techniques improving for some older indications.

Most aspects of the mode of action have not been explained. The major properties of DMSO are:

(1) Relief of pain of injured or inflamed tissue. High concentration of DMSO applied to a nerve will delay conduction and eventually produce a block, but this has not been demonstrated in humans.

(2) A mild anti-inflammatory agent in animals, even with large doses. It partially or completely blocks certain auto immune connective tissue reactions like Freund's Adjuvant Arthritis and PPLO Arthritis in rats.

(3) It passes through skin without producing significant damage —a unique property. Other small molecules can pass through skin with DMSO to achieve a high concentration at a local site without systemic effect and undesirable dose-related side effects. Absorption may vary from one individual to another.

(4) It inhibits the growth of a wide variety of organisms in 20–40 per cent concentration. It is bacteriocidal to some organisms. Clinically, we have not observed spread of infections when DMSO was applied. However, DMSO should be used with caution in disorders when infection is, or may be present.

(5) Solvent effect on collagen has been demonstrated in scleroderma.

CLINICAL INFORMATION

INDICATIONS FOR USE

At the present time the main areas of use seem to be in 1. Orthopedics, 2. Rheumatology, 3. Surgery, and 4. Dermatology.

I. Acute inflammatory or traumatic conditions: 1. Acute bursitis, 2. Acute low back strains, 3. Acute soft tissue injuries, 4. Acute neck strains, and 5. Burns.

II. Chronic conditions–Rheumatology: 1. Ostheoarthritis of a) knees, and b) small joints of hand, 2. Rheumatoid arthritis, 3. Scleroderma and other connective tissue diseases.

III. Surgery: 1. Thoracic, 2. Abdominal, 3. Rectal and Pelvic, and 4. Orthopedic.

IV. Dermatology: 1. Acne and 2. Psoriasis.

EXPERIENCE WITH DMSO IN SPECIFIC DISORDERS

The total clinical experience to date with DMSO supplied by the Merck Sharp & Dohme Research Laboratories involves approximately 4,000 patients. The duration of treatment has ranged from a single application to daily administration up to 18 months.

ACUTE BURSITIS—The largest clinical trials have been in this disorder. In the majority of patients, decreased pain and increased range of motion has been observed in about 30 to 60 minutes. Relief lasts 2 to 6 hours, and usually the intensity of pain is not as severe when it returns. 70 per cent and 90 per cent seem to work equally well. 70 per cent causes less skin reaction.

ACUTE LOW BACK STRAINS—Relief of pain and discomfort has been spectacular in some cases. Accurate diagnosis is essential. In the majority of patients decreased pain and increased range of motion has been observed in 30–60 minutes.

ACUTE TRAUMATIC DISORDERS—Strains, sprains, contusions, athletic injuries, industrial injuries and other traumatic situations have usually responded quite dramatically to DMSO. DMSO has masked a few fractures, so x-ray diagnosis in most cases is advisable.

ACUTE NECK STRAINS (whiplash)—Wide area application has given good results.

OSTEOARTHRITIS—DMSO applied to osteoarthritis of the knees has produced a favorable response after 4 to 6 weeks of daily administration. Transient relief may occur before this time. Increased mobility and general ability to walk and perform tasks without pain has been remarkable in some cases.

RHEUMATOID ARTHRITIS—DMSO seems less effective here than

in certain other diseases. Grades 3 and 4 responded only partially after prolonged administration. DMSO probably would be an adjunct to other forms of therapy.

SCLERODERMA—DMSO has produced considerable softening of the skin and subcutaneous tissue and general improvement in a number of scleroderma patients. Almost all cases have shown some improvement. The concentration should be increased to 90 per cent or higher as skin tolerance increases.

BURNS—DMSO relieves pain in burns, including sunburn, in 10–30 minutes.

NEURALGIAS AND PAIN SYNDROMES—A wide variety of pain syndromes have responded to DMSO. In tic douloureux, or trigeminal neuralgia, some but not all patients have obtained benefit. Treatment must be over a long time. The pain relief may not be permanent. Herpes Zoster has responded most favorably.

ISCHEMIC AND VARICOSE ULCERS—Some chronic ulcers that have not responded to other forms of therapy have improved with DMSO.

DUPUYTREN'S CONTRACTURE—Long-term administration has caused some improvement in fibrous scar contractures. 90 per cent is recommended.

PEYRONIE'S DISEASE—In a few patients so far treated, decreased size of the plaques and straightening of the penis has been noted.

REMOVAL OF CASTS—More rapid mobilization of joints that have been in casts has been observed.

THROMBOPHLEBITIS—Some pain relief when DMSO is applied over thrombosed vessels.

GOUT—There have been a few cases of dramatic relief of pain and general improvement.

VARICOSE VEINS—Relief of pain from varicose veins has been observed.

SINUSITIS—A dilute solution to the nasal mucosa has resulted in the discharge of a great deal of infected material from the sinuses and relief of pain.

SURGERY—After thoracotomies, cholecystectomies and hemorrhoidectomies, 5 to 15 cc. dose 3–4 times/day, results have been very good.

ACNE—There have been some encouraging results. Long term administration has been necessary.

PSORIASIS—Pilot studies are underway. Results may be better with DMSO/Decadron than with DMSO alone. Long term therapy is necessary.

ADMINISTRATION AND DOSAGE

At the present time investigational use of DMSO is limited to cutaneous and mucous membrane administration.

DMSO should be used alone and not mixed with other drugs until toxicity studies with such mixtures have been completed.

DOSAGE—The volume of DMSO to be used in most disorders such as a shoulder or a knee is 8–10 cc., applied three times a day in acute and twice a day in chronic situations, with a cotton-tipped applicator or cotton ball.

The gel formulation, measured in a teaspoon or other suitable container, should be rubbed into the skin with the hand until a thin film results.

Small joints of the hand may be simply dipped into a solution, or it can be applied with an applicator or cotton ball.

Clothing should not be allowed to touch the area until the skin has dried for 30 to 40 minutes. One must be especially careful with synthetic fibers like Orlon and Rayon, since DMSO is a good solvent for these materials.

CONCENTRATIONS—Experience indicates that 90 per cent is not well tolerated on the face and neck, and in almost every case 70 per cent should be used. 70 per cent in most other situations is as satisfactory as with 90 per cent. Where 90 per cent has proved too irritating, start with 50 per cent and then increase to 70 per cent as tolerance increases.

RECOMMENDED AREA OF APPLICATION FOR SPECIFIC DISORDERS

ACUTE BURSITIS—Start just below the ear on the involved side and carry over the shoulder halfway down the arm, and anteriorly to the mid-clavicular line and down to the nipple, and on the back to cover the scapula.

ACUTE TRAUMATIC DISORDERS—(Example: Ankle sprain)—Application to the entire foot and halfway up the leg.

ACUTE LOW BACK STRAINS—Start at the twelfth rib or just below the rib cage, in a band approximately 12 inches wide down to and including the coccyx, and laterally over both sacroilian areas.

ACUTE NECK STRAINS—The entire back of neck from the base of the skull down to and including the shoulders, and on the sides to cover strenocleidomastoid muscle.

OSTEOARTHRITIS OF THE KNEES—From six inches above to six inches below the patella all the way around the leg.

OSTEOARTHRITIS OF HANDS—Entire hand up to wrist with about 5 cc.

RHEUMATOID ARTHRITIS OF THE HANDS—Entire hand and halfway up the forearm or a similar wide area.

SCLERODERMA—Wide area application. The dose has been as high as 100 cc. and in a few instances almost total body application has been attempted. Therapy must be continued and the concentration increased to 90 per cent.

TIC DOULOUREUX OR TRIGEMINAL NEURALGIA—If possible, apply to the entire side of the head and neck affected.

A. *Acute Inflammatory or Traumatic Situations*
Some pain relief usually occurs within one hour. At 2 hours the pain is usually reduced by at least 50 per cent. Continue for three to seven days to assure that the condition does not recur.

B. *Chronic Conditions*
Response has usually been slower and the pain relief from a single or a few applications may be transient. A significant response

may not be obtained until after 4 to 12 weeks of daily administration.

PRECAUTIONS AND CONTRAINDICATIONS

1. DMSO should not be used in infants, children or pregnant patients until adequate toxicity and teratogenic studies have been completed.

2. DMSO should not be applied to skin on which there is any drug or chemical.

3. As with any new drug, DMSO should be used with caution in patients with liver or kidney disease.

4. Some areas of skin such as the face, neck, and axilla are more sensitive to the irritant properties of DMSO than other areas. Also, individuals with blond or red hair seem to react more to the DMSO. The concentration should be reduced to 50 per cent or 70 per cent in these cases. (Note: Dilution of DMSO with water will produce heat. This is not a chemical reaction but only heat of dilution. There is no hazard involved.)

5. If any systemic allergic symptoms develop or there are any signs of general histamine reaction—generalized dermatitis, urticaria, wheal and erythema at sites distant from the original application, lingual edema, asthma, laryngeal edema—the DMSO should be stopped. The area should be washed with water to take off any excess. If appropriate to the clinical situation any other drug to counteract these symptoms (epinepherine, steroids, aminophylline) should be used.

ADVERSE REACTIONS

Approximately 85 per cent of patients experience a typical histamine-type reaction at the site of application, usually transient mild itching and burning and some erythema. This is not considered to be a true adverse reaction to the drug but a typical side effect. A fine vesiculation, occasionally at the site of application, is also usually transient. After prolonged administration, drying, mild wrinkling and occasionally some scaling of the skin is not uncommon. This is no worse than after a mild sunburn.

A few cases of generalized dermatitis have occurred. This is usually a wheal and erythema reaction of a histamine type occurring at sites distant from the area of application. Rarely may this generalized dermatitis be so severe. The drug should be discontinued if a generalized dermatitis develops.

Rarely, serious or potentially serious hypersensitivity reactions may occur. One fatal reaction has been reported in a patient who continued to receive the drug after signs of extreme sensitivity developed.

There has also been a report of laryngeal edema of a mild degree in one patient.

Other unusual reactions have included hypotension in a few patients.

A few cases of mild paresthesias have been noted. Re-evaluation of most of these cases has shown that these were in patients with a strong emotional overlay. Elimination of this type of patient from the clinical studies has greatly reduced this type of reaction.

Some patients have noted a tranquilizing or sedative effect. In most cases this has not been severe enough to warrant concern.

Sedation may occur more in elderly patients with cerebral arteriosclerosis. In the younger individual it occurs more often before meals. It may occur after the first application and, if it is observed, the patient should be cautioned about driving or pursuits that may harm himself or others. Some patients have noted an apparent potentiation of sedatives like barbiturates or alcohol. These findings have not been observed in the laboratory.

Some patients have a garlic or oyster odor on their breath after topical administration of DMSO. There have been a few cases of mild nausea. All of these effects have disappeared when the drug was discontinued.

ABSORPTION, EXCRETION AND METABOLISM OF DMSO—DMSO is absorbed through the skin and distributed through all tissues. The half life of DMSO in serum is about 48 hours. DMSO is excreted primarily in the urine, with some converted to dimethyl sulfide (DMS) which is excreted via the lungs.

Some of the DMSO is converted to dimethyl sulfone (DMSOO) which is excreted in urine over a period of days (1–15) after a single application. There is possibility of a gradual buildup of DMSO and dimethyl sulfone (DMSOO) in blood and tissue with repeated and prolonged administration.

CLINICAL TOXICOLOGY

Laboratory data are being accumulated on patients who have received DMSO by topical application to the skin for a period of one month up to 18 months. To date, there has been no evidence that DMSO produced kidney or liver damage or any significant or permanent changes in blood chemistries after topical application to the skin. No significant changes in the peripheral blood picture have been noted.

Blood chemistries have been followed on a large number of patients, and these have not shown significant changes.

If a patient is to be treated with DMSO for more than one week, pre-treatment laboratory studies should be obtained and repeated at four weeks and then at three months, and every three months thereafter as long as therapy is continued. No laboratory tests are usually necessary for acute conditions in which treatment is contemplated for less than two weeks.

Earlier studies included oral administration of the drug. This route of administration is not being investigated at the present time. (Oral and parenteral studies may be initiated at a later date.) These patients received 30 to 60 ml. per day orally for a period of two weeks, and weight loss from 5 to 10 pounds was noted in 50 per cent of the patients. This may have been from loss of appetite.

Although these changes in liver or renal function have only been observed following administration of large doses of DMSO orally, it is recommended that patients with liver or kidney disease be excluded from clinical trials with DMSO applied topically.

I was in Portland, Oregon, September 9, 1965, and I met Jacob and Rosenbaum at the latter's office. We were going to lunch at the nearby Roses's—a popular restaurant run by Ed's mother-in-law, a little like Lindy's in New York but with popular prices and better food.

Both doctors looked tense, as we walked the hundred or so steps to the restaurant. Finally, Stanley mentioned it: "It had to happen sooner or later," he said sadly. "A patient died from medication—DMSO."

"All drugs are toxic," Rosenbaum said. "Why should DMSO be different from the rest?"

At this point, Jacob and Rosenbaum had only the sketchiest information. Someone on the telephone that morning said that someone else had read of the tragedy in the *Wall Street Journal*.

"It was a lady in Ireland," Jacob said. "As I get it, her tongue swelled and she choked. Apparently an allergic reaction to DMSO."

I was to hear for many years—and I am still hearing—about "the lady in Ireland" who died of a reaction to DMSO. Spokesmen for the FDA frequently allude to "the lady in Ireland" to justify their banning DMSO.

The story, written by William M. Carley, a staff reporter, appeared under the two-column headline:

DMSO MAY HAVE CAUSED DEATH OF WOMAN
MAKERS OF 'WONDER' DRUG WARN DOCTORS

In brief, an unidentified doctor serving an identified drug house (Squibb) had said the woman died after taking DMSO in an approved dosage along with penicillin (which regularly kills quite a few patients each year) and other drugs.

The story said in part:

New York—Drug companies began notifying doctors that DMSO, a so-called "wonder" drug used for pain relief, may have caused the death of a 44-year-old woman being treated with the medication.

The woman, who died three days after application of DMSO began, may have died of an allergic reaction to the substance, according to the warning notice.

The case gives the first indication that DMSO may produce dangerous side effects or allergic reactions.

Doctors cautioned that it hadn't been proved that DMSO caused the death. No autopsy was made. They also said that even if it were proved, the reaction might be so rare that it would still be worthwhile to use the drug in some cases.

Six drug companies are leading intensive investigation of the drug under FDA controls. The six are the Squibb division of Olin Mathieson Chemical Corp., Merck & Co., Syntex Corp., American Home Products Corp., Schering Corp. and Geigy Chemical Co.

Squibb supplied the DMSO used on the woman who died. A Squibb physician said she may have died of an allergic reaction, possibly to DMSO. In letters, the company warned about 100 doctors testing DMSO in the U.S. to halt use of the drug on a patient if allergic reactions showed up.

Merck also sent letters to doctors testing the drug. The company wrote it had learned of the death that was "possibly the result of treatment with DMSO" and also warned doctors to halt DMSO use if a patient showed allergic symptoms.

The Squibb physician gave this account of the death. The

woman, who was living at her home in Ireland, sprained her wrist and knee. Her doctor instructed her to apply DMSO to the skin in those areas. On the first day of medication she developed swelling of the tongue and throat, shortness of breath and difficulty in breathing.

On the second day she applied the drug again and experienced the same reactions. Relatives suggested she call her physician but she decided to wait another day. Some time after visiting her doctor on the third day, she died. The Squibb physician estimated she had applied about 30 milliliters of DMSO, which is in the dosage range that the drug is being tested.

Doctors weren't sure that DMSO caused the allergic reaction and death, however, because other drugs were involved. The woman had previously developed a skin irritation from a hair-removing compound and the irritation developed into an infection. She received five injections of penicillin for the infection and this, plus iodine, cleared it up. The Squibb physician said there wasn't any apparent immediate reaction to the penicillin, but that there may have been a delayed reaction that caused death. Administration of penicillin began June 17 and application of DMSO began July 8.

The Squibb doctor also noted that the woman had been given a prescription for a drug to combat depression five days prior to the beginning of DMSO application. Whether the woman actually took the drug is unknown.

The Squibb report raises several questions: 1) Why the emphasis on DMSO when several other drugs (including some not mentioned in this account) were involved? 2) Why the *Wall Street Journal*? and 3) Was it because inexpensive DMSO was proving superior to many extremely expensive drugs?

On September 22, 1965, Edward H. Nunn, the Crown Zellerbach general manager wired Jacob: "We received at 3 P.M. today a telegram from Mr. George P. Larrick, Commissioner of Food and Drugs, Washington, D.C., stating our exemption for the clinical investigational drug use of dimethyl sulfoxide, IND 1310, has been terminated. The telegram states, 'Administration to human beings should be discontinued and the drug recalled from all clinical investigation.' Pursuant to this termination, we hereby direct that you immediately discontinue all further clinical investigation and return all unused portions of dimethyl sulfoxide to us."

Jacob and Rosenbaum could not regard the FDA's action as more than a bit of bureaucratic finagling—so absurd that it would be forgotten if ignored. Crown's new stern countenance they could have anticipated. For some time, the corporation and its principal officers had seemed jittery. Neither Jacob nor Rosenbaum felt any responsibility toward Crown.

Doomsday for DMSO, however, came about seven weeks later —on November 10, 1965.

Boost, calling from Syntex in Palo Alto, said: "Stanley, it's all over. The Food and Drug Administration has just halted research on dimethyl sulfoxide. They have sent out telegrams notifying the World Health Organization and the Amercian embassies throughout the world."

The spirit drained out of the surgeon. This could mean the end of DMSO, not only in the United States but everywhere.

When Rosenbaum picked up Jacob for a regular weekly drive to Salem, where they would treat Boost's mother, Jacob was still pale, and he seemed on the verge of tears. It was a dreary ride.

"What do you propose to do?" Rosenbaum asked on the return trip.

"Fight," Jacob said. "Naturally. We are doctors and scientists. We have an obligation to our patients and to humanity."

"The FDA can get tough," Rosenbaum reminded him. "And Crown can let us down."

"We'll meet those problems as they arise," Jacob said. His pallor had gone.

The FDA wasted no time in launching a barrage of publicity proclaiming the alleged blinding effects of DMSO. Within a few hours, the news media—domestic and foreign—had all the details, as served up by the FDA's alert corps of press agents.

Predictably, the editorial writers, inspired by the statements of FDA spokesmen and the handouts, thanked heaven that the country once again had been saved from a thalidomide-type debacle. And the radio and TV commentators in their most solemn and sonorous tones did likewise.

In clinics throughout the land doctors reviewed their data to determine whether there was any suggestion of eye damage; they failed to find a single serious defect of any kind which reasonably could be laid to DMSO.

Jacob's patients called to ask, "Is it true that DMSO has made people blind?" He told them he knew of no such evidence. When they asked what they could to continue DMSO treatments, Jacob told them they could write to their Congressmen.

The drug houses did not protest strenuously. In recalling unused DMSO from doctors, Syntex explained:

> The changes observed in the refractive index of the lens in experimental animals—dogs, rabbits, and swine—do not appear to be related to the development of cataracts. In limited studies to date, this change has not been demonstrated in humans treated with dimethyl sulfoxide for prolonged periods of time at relatively high dosages.
>
> In the affected animals, two zones appear in the lens, a central zone of variable diameter and a surrounding peripheral zone. The two zones are distinctly separate. It appears that this change represents a difference in the refractive index between the two zones, and both areas remain transparent. [Possibly indicating nearsightedness.] Microscopic examinations of sections of the affected eyes reveal no difference between the control and experimental animal.
>
> The changes have been seen in dogs following oral administration of DMSO at all doses tested (1.0 to 40 ml/kg). Similar changes have been seen following topical (dermal) application of DMSO to dogs, rabbits and swine. The degree of these changes appears to be dose-related.

Crown Zellerbach first called Jacob demanding that he stop

advising patients to protest. Then Crown followed with this telegraphic reminder:

> This is to confirm our conversation and understanding on the telephone today to the effect that Crown Zellerbach Corporation is unalterably opposed to your advising any patients or others that they appeal to members of Congress or any other government officials, Food and Drug Administration and pharmaceutical companies' decision to suspend investigational use of DMSO. You agreed you would not further encourage any patients or others to pursue this course of action and will attempt to contact those you have previously talked to to persuade them from this course of action.

True to his promise, Jacob contacted those he earlier had enlisted and asked them to call off their protests.

Meanwhile, volunteers were mobilizing spontaneously in rebellion against law and order as promulgated by the Food and Drug Administration. They included patients who felt the FDA had consigned them to pain, and disease, and death; and they were led by doctors who had seen the healing effects of DMSO and who had decided the FDA was wrong.

This is the way Jacob and Rosenbaum later reconstructed events:

The two agents of the Food and Drug Administration—let us call them oo6 and oo9—were polite, businesslike. Jacob and the medical school administrators offered complete co-operation.

They began photocopying Jacob's files late in November 1965, and they continued busily through most of December. At times they would ask Jacob questions, and he would answer them. As time wore on, the agents became less friendly; their questions became more pointed; their comments were sharply critical of the record keeping.

Then one day, their picture taking took them to the animal care department—where they had no permission to explore. The director, Allan Rogers, protested to Joseph Adams, the Assistant Dean for Institutional Relations, who promptly summoned the two men to his office. One of them opened his camera and took out and destroyed the film. Mollified, the medical school officers then gave the FDA agents permission to go ahead and take pictures of the animal housing quarters.

The week before Christmas the agents asked to examine case records and a DMSO distribution file. Jacob gave them the go-ahead. Two days later, on December 21, 1965, Jacob said, he found the agents, with characteristic industry, photocopying his personal correspondence.

"Look," Jacob said to 006 and 009, "I know that this may be an honest mistake, but before you proceed further with the files I want your assurance that every photocopy so far made will be destroyed. Then let me know what you want, and I'll get it for you."

Jacob said 009 told him that since he had used government equipment and did the photocopying on government time, they couldn't give away government property.

Something shook Jacob's trust in these two men. The same agents had destroyed the government's film when they were caught taking pictures of the animal care facilities on government time.

"Are you kidding?" Jacob asked.

"No," 009 answered.

Bill Zimmerman, Assistant Dean for Business Affairs, called the FDA district director in Seattle and filed a protest on behalf of the medical school.

Rosenbaum entered his office one morning a half-hour late and somewhat tense. He had just rescued a patient in cardiac arrest, but he still wasn't sure the patient would make it. His waiting room was full.

Two surprise guests—009 and 012—were showing the receptionist their credentials. Because you don't keep important government representatives waiting, Rosenbaum took them into the consultation room, where they repeated the story told Jacob earlier.

Rosenbaum said the agents had a sense of humor. One of them said with disarming charm, "Look, we have no guns—no hidden microphones." And amid their laughter, both of them held up their arms, so anyone could see they were telling the truth. Rosenbaum gave them the records of about 200 of his 600 or 700 patients, sent them on their way, and he went to work on his impatient patients.

The constitutionality of the FDA regulation which says that FDA agents may enter a physician's office and inspect the records of patients on an experimental drug isn't above challenge. Even the insurance carriers' rights to invade patients' privacy may be a passing privilege.

Political figures, businessmen and beggars have secrets on the doctors' cards to which FDA plainclothes police were demanding access. An old venereal disease, marital troubles, a defective child or sibling, a chronic illness—these are among the confessions patients entrust to their physicians' files.

The FDA agents didn't bother to advise Rosenbaum of his rights: to remain silent, to have legal counsel.

Rosenbaum, worried, dialed Norman B. Kobin, attorney-at-law.

"You mean these agents demanded to see your patients' records? And you obliged them?" Kobin was incredulous.

"Yes," Rosenbaum faltered. "You see—"

"The agents violated your fundamental rights as a citizen," Kobin stormed. "And they breached a sacred doctor-patient relationship."

When the FDA inspectors returned a few days later for more records, Rosenbaum took them into an examining room. There he introduced them to Kobin's son, Chuck, also an attorney.

Chuck Kobin switched on a tape recorder. "Just so there won't be any misunderstanding," he explained. "Now, please explain your mission."

"For a half-hour, the agents hemmed and hawed," Rosenbaum said later. "When Mr. Kobin told them they were violating a patient-physician ethic by recording the names of patients, the agents said they would block out the names. Mr. Kobin advised them that he wanted, in writing, an explanation from their superior in Seattle."

Two days later one of the inspectors called from Seattle to complain that Rosenbaum was delaying the work of the FDA. Rosenbaum suggested the inspector talk to his attorney and pointed out that Crown Zellerbach and Merck had duplicate records of his DMSO treatments. A few days later both inspectors again appeared in Rosenbaum's office and gave him a slip of paper threatening to invoke a federal regulation unless he surrendered the records.

"What regulation?" Rosenbaum asked. The inspectors said they didn't know.

That was the last Rosenbaum saw of them.

For several reasons, Stanley Jacob was reluctant to do what his common sense told him to do—hire a lawyer.

First of all, he couldn't believe his government wished him ill. Litigation meant time away from his work, a destructive distraction from his beloved DMSO.

And then there was the overpowering burden of expense. Only Jacob knew it, but he was desperately broke and going deeper into debt with each passing day.

Maybe if he didn't think about it, his trouble with the FDA would go away. The FDA would not go away, however.

And so Stanley Jacob asked Ed Rosenbaum to introduce him to Norm Kobin.

In the middle of the investigation, Ed Rosenbaum had a caller. "I work for the FDA," he said. "But I can't stomach what they're doing to you."

This is the way Rosenbaum relayed the agent's account to me:

Two weeks after DMSO testing was stopped, almost every FDA inspector was called back to Washington for a briefing. It was the biggest call-back of inspectors that ever occurred. The inspectors were told that there was serious question as to whether the FDA had been right in stopping DMSO because of toxicity. They were told to go out in the field and find some "pigeons."

The inspectors were interested in proving that the DMSO investigators had been dishonest. They were also very interested in finding the names of any patients who had had side effects or bad results and who would testify to the damage before congressional committees.

The purpose was to try the original investigators in the press.

There was considerable jockeying within the agency for positions of power and for promotions. Everyone was jealous of Dr. Kelsey, who had received a medal for stopping thalidomide. And everyone was in hopes that they had another thalidomide or krebiozen story to glorify the FDA and win promotions.

"He told me the smartest thing I could do was get myself a lawyer," Rosenbaum said.

Rosenbaum called Herschler and asked if Crown Zellerbach would provide a lawyer. Herschler seemed to think this would be in Crown's interest; but the next day Herschler called to say Crown refused. And neither would Crown associate itself in any way with Jacob and Rosenbaum, he added.

Rosenbaum had another visit from the friendly FDA agent. "He told me that FDA inspectors, in the guise of having me sign a permit to examine a chart had me sign a blank sheet of paper," Rosenbaum told me.

He quoted his informant as saying, "The inspectors are down in the office now, laughing and wondering how to use your signature." He told Rosenbaum that the inspectors were copying Jacob's personal correspondence, and he gave Rosenbaum a copy of one personal letter of Jacob's which had nothing whatsoever to do with DMSO, Rosenbaum said.

At this point, Jacob and Rosenbaum decided they had better defend themselves.

Part Two

"I think I need help," Jacob said. "I should tell you, however, that I don't have a lot of money."

"More than money is involved here," the lawyer said. "We won't worry about it."

So Norman B. Kobin, attorney-at-law, took the case.

Kobin, a middle-aged, easygoing man, took the initiative. He wrote a letter to the FDA district director in Seattle protesting their agents' prying into Jacob's private and professional affairs on matters that had nothing to do with DMSO.

Kobin, as attorney for both Jacob and Rosenbaum, hoped to stop the harassment without triggering reprisals.

"The two FDA agents made an inspection and search of records belonging to Dr. Jacob far beyond the scope of the authority given," Kobin charged. "Unauthorized photocopies were made and taken from the premises." He demanded that the FDA return the photocopies forthwith and that "instructions be issued to the two agents and to all other agents of the FDA not to disclose any information gained as a result of this unauthorized search and seizure."

"This letter is directed to Seattle in order to afford your office the opportunity to correct this matter at the local level," Kobin conceded. "Should satisfactory compliance with this matter not be forthcoming within the next 10 days, we shall have no alternative but to take such steps on Dr. Jacob's behalf as may seem appropriate."

The answer to Kobin's challenge came from Washington, not Seattle. It was addressed to Jacob, not Kobin. It was signed by James Lee Goddard, M.D., the FDA Commissioner, who said he had been told that Jacob had expressed concern about the FDA's possession of the photocopies. Goddard wrote that it was his view that, with "very few exceptions," the copies of the documents were pertinent to the FDA investigation of DMSO; and he wanted to meet with Jacob to discuss which of the documents Jacob felt should not have been in the FDA's hands.

Kobin found little satisfaction with the FDA's response, particularly with the commissioner's argument that in effect, his police had honored Jacob's constitutional rights "with very few exceptions."

Ten days after he became Commissioner of the Food and Drug Administration, Goddard had received Kobin's note. Energetic, ambitious, deeply dedicated to law enforcement, a self-declared "activist," Goddard may have regarded the incident as heaven-sent. He was about to ask Congress for police powers which never before had been exercised in the United States over a category of citizens—scientists and physicians—for whom the law had been lax. The case of this Oregon scientist and the ridiculous panacea he was distributing far and wide may have seemed to offer perfect support for the FDA's position.

Goddard did not wait for Jacob to move. He presented the case against DMSO on March 9, 1966, at a hearing before the House of Representatives Fountain Subcommittee on Drug Safety, more formally called the Subcommittee on Intergovernmental Relations of the House Committee on Government Operations. Subcommittee people made no secret of their admiration for this keen-eyed, tense, lean civil servant; they liked his ready grasp of the agency's aims and the way he handled himself and his group of aides, whom he played as though they were chess pieces:

Mr. William W. "Billy" Goodrich, a lawyer with the title Assistant General Counsel, Department of Health, Education, and Welfare. Many considered him the architect of the latter day FDA;

Dr. Frances O. Kelsey, his Chief of the Investigational Drug Branch, who had been given a gold medal by President Kennedy for supposedly keeping thalidomide out of the United States;

Dr. Joseph F. Sadusk, Jr., Medical Director, whom some had considered heir apparent to the commissionership until Goddard came along; and

Dr. Robert M. Hodges and Dr. Harold Anderson, a couple of bureau wheelhorses.

Goddard opened and introduced himself to the subcommittee with a background sheet and an FDA press release on President Johnson's announcement of his appointment. The data included: born, April 24, 1923, in Alliance, Ohio; married; three children; *EDUCATION:* Warren, Ohio, high school; Mount Union College, Washington and Lee University, Temple University, and, for his M.D. in 1949, George Washington University School of Medicine. He was in the Army 1943–46. As an officer of the U. S. Public Health Service during and after his internship and with other government bureaus in 1949 until he became FDA Commissioner on January 17, 1966, he had served traineeships in the New York State Department of Health in Albany, the Harvard School of Public Health and the District Health Department in Chapel Hill, N.C. He was a member of a dozen medical groups; and under *"Awards"* he had listed three earned in 1962: the John Jeffries, the P.H.S. Meritorious Service Medal and the Distinguished Service Award of the Federal Aviation Agency.

In the seventeen years since he had won his M.D., Goddard had been in private practice a total of fourteen months. With this background, he was now to wield unprecedented, some charged almost dictatorial, power over the practice of medicine in the United States.

Goddard himself outlined to the Fountain Subcommittee the requirements, under the 1962 Kefauver-Harris Amendments to the Pure Food and Drug Act: in Phases One and Two of testing, drug houses must present complete data on a proposed drug—chemical, biological, source, strength, purity. They must identify those who will test the preparation in the laboratory, give their qualifications, and list the facilities. With animal data compiled, Phase Three—final clinical trials—may be undertaken; this calls for detailed physical and chemical examination of subjects given the drug, careful recording of data, and periodic reports. Sponsors could not advertise or sell the drug while under study.

Goddard said the FDA retained the right to order an investigation discontinued if there were false or incomplete data, deviation from the plan, signs of ill effects, lack of effectiveness, inadequacy of facilities or controls, elements of commercialization, or indication that the plan is unreasonable.

"I fail to see how anyone could disagree with the purpose of the regulations," Goddard said.

The committee members nodded agreement with the bright, earnest new commissioner.

Goddard's testimony before the Fountain Subcommittee on March 9, 1966, was a product not only of his own long experience in bureaucracy but also of the genius of Billy Goodrich, the FDA's playmaker, author of many of the statements read, and the commissioner's coach throughout the session.

Goddard testified: "I am instructing the formulation of clear internal policy and procedure guidelines for the performance of adequate surveillance over the conduct of clinical investigations under IND's. We believe such attention will improve the quality of performance and the probative value of research. *We have a delicate problem in investigating the investigator.* [Emphasis mine.] Scientific personnel are not accustomed to being ques-

84

tioned by regulatory agencies. But some investigations will have to be made and when it becomes necessary to do so every effort will be made to minimize misunderstanding."

To minimize any of the subcommittee's misunderstanding of the need to lend his bureau a few of the citizen's liberties, he outlined briefly the FDA's charges against Crown, Jacob and DMSO.

Goddard said:

In October 1963, a plan for the clinical investigation was filed. Review showed the animal studies to be so incomplete as to warrant only the most limited of use in human beings, and the firm was advised that approval extended only to external application to the skin of DMSO alone, not combined with any substance other than water, and limited as to factors of duration and concentration.

The firm made arrangements to license the use of DMSO under their patents to six large drug firms, each of which in turn filed the required plan of investigation. We have found that in the next 2 years, one or more of the firm's investigators:

(1) Disseminated glowing reports of the speculated value of the drug in a wide variety of conditions.

(2) Had performed some further animal studies which, when submitted, were believed by them to warrant gross expansion of the clinical studies although no such expansion was justified by the studies.

(3) Distributed the drug to many physicians who wanted it simply for purposes of therapy, without exercising any of the safeguards necessary to clinical investigation, and without many of these physicians being listed as investigators.

(4) Exported substantial quantities of the drug without regard to the requirement of the law or the reporting requirement of the investigational plan.

(5) Failed to report new investigators and new procedures of use beyond topical application until long after the studies were underway.

(6) Never initiated the comprehensive animal studies which had been originally requested by FDA as a basis for Phase Three investigation.

85

(7) Encouraged use of the drug by oral administration, injection, bladder irrigation, application to mucous membranes, application to the eyes, use for conditions not specified in the plan, and use in combination with a wide variety of other drugs, for which conditions there had been no suitable safety data supplied.

Speculation and enthusiastic promotion both to the profession and to the public was substituted for scientific inquiry and deliberate evaluation of evidence. This resulted in unwarranted distribution for use as a therapeutic agent by many physicians, before the animal or human studies had established either safety or efficacy.

Plainly, the plans submitted to us did not cover what was actually being done, nor did the data available to us or to the sponsors provide an adequate basis for the broad-ranging distribution of this investigational new drug.

Goddard mentioned that the FDA had warned one of the drug companies in June 1965 about illegal use of DMSO. He told of the refractive changes in the lens of the eyes of some test animals and the suspension of all investigational use of DMSO on November 11, 1965.

"I have, however, permitted continued use for a few investigators to administer to specific patients—about 50—having the conditions scleroderma, tic douloureux, Raynaud's phenomena, and multiple sclerosis," Goddard said.

Goddard served notice that "we are investigating possible criminal violations." This remark was headlined throughout the United States.

It fell to Sadusk to justify the FDA's program.

Sadusk could be—and was—fairly specific about the toxicity detected in animal studies: the changes in the refractive index in dogs fed DMSO and in rabbits painted with DMSO. He neglected to point out, however, that 100 times the human dose had been given the animals.

It is noteworthy that Sadusk at one point could complain that "very extensive publicity appeared in the popular press, representing DMSO to be a wonder drug for the treatment of a variety of diseases" and a few minutes later tell of the FDA's resort to the press release to warn "of the dangers of DMSO" to the human eye, another charge without any proof.

Sadusk cited—but did not identify—reports suggesting a "probable relationship" of DMSO to "impaired vision of a vague type," "decreasing vision," "pain in one eye," etc.

He said that systemic allergic reactions had been reported "with at least one death." Yes, the lady in Ireland.

Sadusk submitted a catalogue of "Adverse Reactions to DMSO" which he said had been reported; but he neglected to say by whom, or where, or when, or how. And nobody asked. The complaints included:

SKIN—damage to the mucous membrane of the mouth and sloughing at the treated area (four cases);

BLOOD—monocytosis and leukopenia (four cases);

CARDIOVASCULAR—congestive heart failure (one case) and tachycardia, or pounding of the heart (two cases);

LUNG—pneumonitis (two cases), shortness of breath (two cases);

LIVER—hepatitis, "although there does not appear to be a cause-effect relationship" (three cases);

CENTRAL NERVOUS SYSTEM—headache, vertigo, drowsiness (fifteen cases), severe mental confusion (one case);

GASTROINTESTINAL—mostly mild, nausea with or without vomiting (apparently related to garlic taste or odor) (thirty-four cases); and transient GI bleeding (one instance).

"There have been a small number of reports evaluated as not cause related, of cerebrovascular accidents, myocardial infarction, depression, mental confusion, possible abnormal liver function, panmyocarditis, and gastrointestinal bleeding occurring in patients using DMSO," Sadusk testified.

Present at the Fountain subcommittee session the next day were FDA administrators, doctors and press agents, and six representatives of four drug houses (Wyeth, Squibb, Geigy and Merck Sharp & Dohme).

But there wasn't anybody there to defend Stanley Jacob or ask for proof that DMSO was harming and killing people.

Of the more than 70,000 patients enumerated by the FDA at the hearing as having been treated with DMSO on IND's issued to fifteen sponsors other than Crown Zellerbach (Maxwell Abramson, M.D., Ayerst, Geigy, Robert E. Gosselin, M.D., Eli Lilly, Merck, Chas. Pfizer, Procter & Gamble, Sandoz, Schering Corp., Arnold Seligman, M.D., Squibb, Syntex, White Labs and Wyeth Labs) not a single one had been invited to testify as to whether DMSO did him good or ill.

After reading newspaper accounts of the hearing, Jacob fired off this telegram to Fountain:

If the newspaper reports of Dr. Goddard's testimony before your committee are correct, he has done a disservice to himself, his agency and the American people. According to all scientific evidence available, Dr. Goddard's statements of eye damage in man are simply and absolutely not true.

Neither Fountain nor his committee acknowledged the telegram.

Shortly after the Fountain Subcommittee hearings, Sadusk quit the FDA. He worked briefly as Professor of Medicine at Johns Hopkins before following the custom of many former FDA officials—taking a job with the food or drug industry. Sadusk became Vice President for Medical Affairs with Parke, Davis and Company in Detroit.

A few weeks after retiring—on May 17, 1966—he submitted an article, "Drugs and the Public Safety," to the *Annals of Internal Medicine* which was particularly eloquent in what it didn't say. It didn't mention Goddard, for example, although it did praise the "highly dedicated public servants, both medical and nonmedical, both scientific and regulatory," with whom he had worked.

88

Perhaps more pointedly, he paid tribute to "the skillful leadership and guidance which Commissioner Emeritus George Larrick gave to the Administration."

To warn the medical profession of imminent danger—and, one might speculate, possibly in contrition for his own role in the FDA—he wrote:

No one can deny that the provisions of the Federal Food, Drug and Cosmetic Act and its amendments are in the public interest and promote drug safety to a degree not surpassed anywhere in the world. But it must be recognized—and this I cannot stress too strongly—that the provisions of these drastic and far-reaching amendments should be administered in a scientific and flexible manner. An overly strict interpretation and application of the legal and regulatory language of the recent amendments could stifle the development and production of new drugs.

The Food and Drug Administration must arrive at decisions on the basis of a consensus of informal medical opinion, both within and outside the Agency. And above all, the government has an obligation under the law to fully inform the practicing physician on the efficacy and safety of drugs but not to go beyond this point. To tie the hands of the doctor by dogmatic directives in the labeling on the use of a drug, to overemphasize adverse animal data without clinical confirmation, or to stress adverse experiences without a reasonable degree of certainty of a cause-effect relationship is unjustifiable. I hope that all practicing physicians will demand for their patients the privilege and right to prescribe that drug which in their opinion is the best drug to be used at the time of treatment and under the circumstances which surround that treatment. It must be the physician, as the patient's doctor, who maintains the ultimate responsibility for the treatment of his patient.

In the same article, Sadusk berated the press for having quoted some scientists' fears that "the pill" to prevent pregnancy was not proved safe, that, for one thing, it might cause thrombophlebitis.

"This is a matter on which there has been much loose talk and speculation, and for which highly sophisticated procedures will be required to completely clarify the matter," he wrote. He said that with 5,000,000 American women taking the pill, it was surprising that many thousands more cases of thrombophlebitis had not been reported due to natural causes. "It is sad to note that many women using these drugs have been unnecessarily alarmed by biased and misleading articles appearing in the lay press and prepared by certain self-appointed experts. It should be the duty of the press to stress conservatism and scientific accuracy in reporting, particularly on matters of drug safety."

While Sadusk's statement was designed to quiet fears, it also tended to promote sales of the pill. Inadvertently, of course. The Merck Manual of 1966, a standard medical reference, and later, the AMA Drug Evaluations—1971 warned of an enhanced risk of thromboembolic disease associated with the pill in British and American studies. The pill was found also to increase the chance of hypertension and anemia, as well as clots, in women and monster offspring in mice. Sadusk wrote his paper well before he joined Parke, Davis, which happens to produce a contraceptive called Norlestrin, and, as he might put it, his paper and his new job probably are not "cause-effect related."

Many months after he had entered industry, I wrote to Sadusk and asked how he then felt about DMSO's toxicity. He said he had had no further contact with the drug since leaving Washington, and he added, "It may be by now that the FDA has sufficient early experimental data to arrive at a new stand."

The FDA, however, was doing business at the same old stand. In January 1968, with a growing disaster having overtaken the nation's introduction of new drugs, the FDA relaxed its rules somewhat, for all drugs but two—LSD and DMSO.

The Fountain subcommittee session served to establish Goddard as a tough commissioner and the threat of investigation as a powerful bureaucratic weapon to keep the profession, the drug industry and the public in line.

A month after Goddard had tested his authority and found it functional before the Fountain Subcommittee, he distributed a note to "Dear Mr. Chemical Supplier," "to ask your help" in the problem of hallucinogenic drugs. He warned, in closing: "Failure to take action to determine legitimate use of these chemicals may result in unnecessary investigations of your activities and possible regulatory action."

Ten days later, Goddard admonished doctors in a luncheon address at the annual meeting of the American Society of Internal Medicine to practice better medicine and assume their responsibilities. "The Food and Drug Administration is a third party in the practice of medicine," he said. He urged his audience to consider the FDA's "recent experience with DMSO."

He was even more hard-boiled with the drug industry and with those who wrote the advertising. He charged industry executives with "excesses in advertising," "misleading statements," "an overabundance of information available to the physician," in the industry's free books, periodicals, direct mail letters and other means of reaching the doctors. Some editorial writers charged that Goddard was following the familiar course toward imposing censorship.

And more and more commentators asserted that the role of the FDA, "the third party in medicine," had become that of Big Brother.

Goddard continued to pay his visits to congressional committees, each time with new success . . . and more power.

The generous gift of police powers awarded to Goddard was not inspired solely by the thalidomide horror, or the abuses of DMSO. The most impelling force, from the public's point of view at least, was the drive against so-called "dangerous drugs," the ghastly stuff that was turning an entire generation of youngsters into killers, arsonists, lunatics, thieves, whores, pimps, gunmen and the walking dead, to satisfy a habit that very few ever could or would shake.

Goddard delineated for the Fountain Subcommittee the authority granted him under the February 1, 1960, Amendments to the Narcotic and Drug Abuse Act. In a statement covering twenty-one pages of single-spaced type, the commissioner said that "the law, as it currently exists, is a good law and one which we feel will enable us to deal with the problems."

He said the amendments:

1. Provide for control over the manufacture of depressant or stimulant drugs and *any drug which contains a substance found by the Secretary of Health, Education, and Welfare to have a potential for abuse because of its depressant or stimulant effect or because of its hallucinogenic effect;*

2. Eliminate the necessity for the Government to prove interstate shipment of them;

3. Require wholesalers and jobbers of the drugs to register with the FDA annually and manufacturers to indicate if they are producing them;

4. Provide that inspectors may:
   a. execute seizures with or without libels of information,
   b. execute and serve arrests and search warrants,
   c. make arrests without warrants in certain cases, and
   d. carry firearms.

"The backbone of our field staff will be composed of criminal investigators," Goddard reported. He said 175 of them—almost all former federal enforcement agents—already had been hired, some as gun toters.

It became evident within the first few months after the FDA had been armed with unprecedented police powers that the agency had scored instant and almost complete success against one "dangerous drug"—DMSO. Most physicians returned their stores of DMSO to the supplier or destroyed them. To have DMSO on the premises was to court raids by FDA agents and criminal prosecution. To continue to use it in the clinic was to invite malpractice suits as well; complainants could cite the FDA attitude to indicate that the physician was in the wrong.

92

Dr. Marvin Paul of Toronto wrote that a big meeting on DMSO should be held in the United States, and Bob Herschler sounded out the New York Academy of Sciences.

The academy responded promptly and positively. It had received similar suggestions from two other independent sources; if a program were prepared the academy would like to consider it.

Everything went well until September, when the FDA suddenly cracked down, charging that the number of doctors testing DMSO for Crown and the number of patients were far greater than the maximum the FDA had permitted.

DMSO, not merely as a new drug but representing a whole new principle in medicine, had attracted physicians and patients in enormous numbers.

Crown's reaction was complete and abject compliance with the FDA's orders. His bosses ordered Herschler to renounce his role with Rosenbaum and Jacob, and this Herschler did. At his age with only a bachelor's degree, new jobs were not easy to find.

The New York Academy is big (almost 27,000 members in fifty states and many foreign countries) and broad (it sponsors meetings for a vast array of scientific disciplines). Its leaders have forged outstanding reputations in their own fields—and many have taken their lickings for creativity. In this organization, stuffy inner politics and do-nothing bureaucracy are at a minimum.

93

Jacob had spent the summer of 1965 writing letters to everyone he knew who had studied DMSO, regardless of whether they thought well or poorly of the compound, and by September he had collected about 100 abstracts on which to propose a program.

Two weeks after Crown Zellerbach was ordered to cease sponsorship of their IND, Dean Baird called Jacob into his office and told him that Crown was bringing great pressure on him to have the New York Academy symposium called off.

"I can't order you to withdraw from leadership in the symposium," Baird told the young surgeon. "I don't regard that as the kind of authority a dean should exercise in a decent and democratic educational institution. My concept of academic freedom, however, does not forbid my advising you that if you go ahead with your present plans, you might embarrass the dean."

Jacob studied his friend. "Under no circumstances would I embarrass the dean," he said, and he repeated: "Under no circumstances."

The dean smiled and said, "But since Dr. Rosenbaum isn't a member of the faculty at this time, I have no control over him. If he were to go ahead and develop the symposium—"

So Ed Rosenbaum went to Two East Sixty-third Street, New York, to negotiate for the proposed meeting. He was amazed at the grasp the academy officers had of the situation and of DMSO. He said that with the large number of papers to be presented, the meeting should run three days, and he would like to hold it seven or eight months hence, in the spring.

The academy officers pointed out that meetings of this size were held usually at the Waldorf Astoria Hotel, which was booked solidly through the spring, and, anyway, other arrangements would take more than one year.

No sooner had Rosenbaum gotten back to Portland than the Academy called Herschler to tell him that, on second thought, the DMSO meeting was so important that a special case was being made for it. If a program could be produced in thirty days, they'd schedule the meeting for March 1966, five months off.

"I wondered about this, and I still do," Rosenbaum said years later. "My guess is that the FDA tried to 'persuade' the New York Academy to call off the meeting. The officers were not men who can be intimidated."

Dean Baird and Jacob (Herschler now was dropping farther and farther into the background) induced Dr. Chauncey Leake of the University of California Medical Center, one of the most respected and powerful figures in medical education, to agree to chair the symposium.

Jacob bent his efforts to seeking negative papers to give the program some balance. It turned out that it was virtually impossible to find knowledgeable scientists who could offer negative or unfavorable reports. He invited Sadusk to send FDA researchers to report; the FDA official replied he would be delighted to oblige, "but rumor has it that the symposium never will be held." His reply came on November 9, 1965—the day before he issued the order banning DMSO research.

When Rosenbaum met Leake in New York he apologized. "We'll understand perfectly if you elect to withdraw now," Rosenbaum said.

"Not a chance, Ed," Leake said. "Let's get to work on the details." They were to present their plan and program to the academy's executive committee for its approval that evening.

Leake asked whether any drug house might pick up the tab for expenses, which, for a meeting of this sort, usually ranged from $20,000 to $50,000.

Rosenbaum's jaw fell. He hadn't thought of this. And with Crown Zellerbach possibly wishing it had never heard of DMSO, there wasn't a chance of support there. The drug houses, too, had lost interest. Both men, deeply discouraged, reported that they would have to call the meeting off after all. The Academy told them, "That won't be necessary. The academy has special funds for this meeting. Don't worry about money."

Leake then received a call from a drug industry leader whom he chooses not to identify. After the conversation, Leake told

Rosenbaum, "My friend asked that we drop plans for the symposium at this time—said it would be very embarrassing to both the drug houses and to the FDA." He decided to call Dean Baird.

After hanging up, Leake turned to Rosenbaum. "Know what Baird said? He said, 'Chauncey, when have you or I, as deans and educators, ever let political or economic considerations compromise the search for scientific truth?' "

Leake didn't talk about it then. As they got up from the dinner table, he said, "Okay, Ed. Let's give the committee our program."

When Leake announced their decision, the committee applauded. "They seemed to have a special interest in this," Rosenbaum said. "It was as though a tenet of scientific morality had been tried—and triumphed."

The March 14, 15 and 16, 1966, symposium under the auspices of the New York Academy of Sciences was held in a large hall of New York's Waldorf Astoria Hotel. More than a thousand researchers came from all parts of the United States and from overseas. After the FDA had cracked down on DMSO, Jacob had written to every person who had submitted an abstract; he said that now that DMSO had been branded toxic and dangerous by the FDA the paper could be withdrawn. No one canceled.

In opening, Dr. Leake jocularly welcomed agents of the Food and Drug Administration and Federal Bureau of Investigation, who were conspicuous by their apathy.

Eighty-two papers had been scheduled, and many additional scientists spoke extemporaneously. With perhaps one exception, Dr. Arthur Ruskin of the FDA, who concentrated on the fine job being done by the FDA and its tolerance of science, the papers reflected virtually unanimous enthusiasm for DMSO's unusual physical, chemical and medical properties. Ruskin's message was, "this symposium is a measure of the freedom of investigation and the responsibilities for it of the United States Government prevailing in this country."

One section was concerned with DMSO's phenomenal ability

to protect living cells and organisms against the damaging and lethal effects of cold and of radiation. Both properties held implications for cancer—DMSO might shield normal tissues in cryosurgery or in supervoltage radiation. Dr. M. J. Ashwood-Smith of Harwell, England, one of the earliest experimenters with DMSO, said he thought the two protective mechanisms might be related.

Papers on DMSO toxicology and pharmacology and others dealing with DMSO's effects on plants and microscopic organisms, told of labeling DMSO with radioactive atoms so that the compound could be traced during its anatomical travels, chemical changes, membrane penetrations, and effects on enzyme systems in nerve cells (giving at least a hypothetical mechanism for its tranquilizing and pain-suppressing effects). Others reported on its influence on coagulation, on antibody, lysosomal and other immune systems, on hormones like cortisone, on a number of skin diseases.

Many speakers confirmed Jacob's early observations in animals and in man. The studies covered a spectrum of diseases probably far greater than any ever before considered in relation to a single drug.

Jacob met an able biochemist, Don C. Wood, Ph.D., then working at Providence Hospital in Portland. Wood, a quiet, self-effacing man, and his junior associates were reporting a long series of tests on rabbits before, during and after administering DMSO to them over many routes. He had made meticulous tests on the chemical composition of the animals' body fluids and blood, the function of organs and tissues during life, and the changes that had come over them at the time of his autopsies.

Jacob needed a first-class biochemist and the time was rapidly approaching when Wood would need a clinician. Some important figures at Providence Hospital were beginning to feel that work with DMSO was a waste of time, and quite possibly dangerous—medically and politically.

One event worth special mention at this time was a paper by

Drs. Eduardo Ramírez of the Laboratorio de Investigaciones Psiquiatrías and Segisfredo Luza of the Cátedra de Psiquiatría, Facultad de Medicina, Universidad Peruana "Cayetano Heredia" —psychiatrists in Lima, Peru. These men reported good results with DMSO in a series of patients with a number of mental diseases.

Ramírez thought that DMSO might have some effect on mental disease because in high doses it seemed to induce fatigue or tranquilization in animals and humans. He felt the sulfur on the phenothiazine molecule lent a tranquilizing effect; that being so, he reasoned, perhaps the sulfur in DMSO would do likewise.

After extensive tests on animals and then on normal human volunteers, Ramírez began injecting 50 per cent or 80 per cent DMSO intramuscularly into patients with acute and chronic schizophrenia, manic-depressive syndrome, alcoholic psychosis, and compulsive and severe anxiety. Control patients were given shock therapy, tranquilizers, sedatives and other standard treatment.

Ramírez reported that of the fourteen acute schizophrenics, every single one was discharged from the hospital within forty-five days after the start of DMSO treatment. Their agitation and other symptoms began to abate after the first few injections. He said that four of the eleven chronic schizophrenics—one of whom had been ill fourteen years—were discharged eventually, and the other seven improved a great deal and were given occupational therapy.

The four diagnosed as manic-depressive psychotics and four others who had alcoholic hallucinations also improved and at length left the hospital. Others with anxiety neuroses also improved and were discharged eventually.

One could find fault with these experiments on the grounds that the control subjects were not given a suitable placebo. Ramírez and Luza could not think of an appropriate placebo. But they did measure the rate of improvement and earlier dismissals. And they were witness to:

The rapid decrease in agitation among catatonic-paranoics;

98

recession of persecution feelings and distrust among the paranoics;

a relatively sudden tendency to communicate and to stay clean and tidy among the chronic schizophrenics;

the wane of obsessions and the return of alertness and interest in events in their environment;

a calmness where there had been restlessness and anxiety.

Ramírez said that aside from the DMSO odor and a few cases of brief insomnia, the patients exhibited no deleterious side effects.

The Peruvians' experiments were considered generally pretty far out.

As the New York Academy sessions were drawing to a close, an FDA agent turned to Ann Sullivan of the Portland *Oregonian*, and said, "DMSO is through."

Ann looked at the man in amazement.

"Where did you ever get that idea?" Miss Sullivan asked.

"My boss told me," the agent answered, according to Miss Sullivan.

The papers presented at the academy sessions were published in a brown paperback volume of 671 pages and several hundred thousand words, *Annals of the New York Academy of Sciences*, Volume 141, Art. 1, *Biological Actions of Dimethyl Sulfoxide.* If it isn't out of print, it can be bought for about fifteen dollars.

Here in a nutshell are some of the points made at the academy meetings:

TOXICITY—Several investigators reported that very high doses of DMSO, often administered by unusual routes, produced clouding of the lens in three animal species. These effects could not be repeated in humans or related species, and some reported they were reversible to a degree.

FREEZING—DMSO overcame the effects in several species.

RADIATION—DMSO strongly protected against lethal x-rays—much moreso than did AET, cysteamine and serotonin (Ashwood-Smith). Moreover, DMSO was effective even when applied only to the skin (F. Golan, Univ. of Miami).

TOXICITY—LD-50 values (the dose needed to kill 50 per cent of the test animals) show DMSO has low systemic toxicity (by oral, intravenous, topical, subcutaneous and intraperitoneal routes) to nine subhuman species. Eye changes appear to be irreversible (Emil R. Smith et al., Mason Research Institute, Worcester, Mass.).

TERATOGENICITY—Injected into chicken eggs in very high doses, DMSO caused birth defects. Pregnant rats, mice and rabbits injected in the belly with high and repeated doses of DMSO occasionally produced defective offspring (F. M. E. Caujolle et al., Toulouse, France). Hamsters were even more susceptible (V. H. Ferm).

PLANTS—DMSO enhanced the phosphorous uptake—and presumably metabolism and growth—of strawberry plants and young pear trees (Ralph Garren, Jr., Oregon State Univ.). DMSO transported bactericides and fungicides into plants and cured or controlled serious infections of peach, plum, apricot, nectarine and other trees (Harry L. Keil, U. S. Dept. of Agriculture, Beltsville, Md.). DMSO transported iron nutrients into citrus trees (C. D. Leonard, Univ. of Florida).

HORMONES—DMSO increased the potency of cortisone-type hormones in cultured cells (D. Berliner, Univ. of Utah).

CANCER AND LEUKEMIA—Organisms frequently found in cancer and leukemia patients and suspected as a cause of cancer stopped growing when exposed to 25 per cent DMSO (F. Seibert et al., Mound Park Hospital Foundation, St. Petersburg). DMSO killed leukemic cells more readily than normal cells growing in the same culture (Robert Schrek et al., V. A. Hospital, Hines, Ill.). DMSO neither speeded nor slowed the growth of cancer cells implanted in the rabbit belly (James R. Armstrong, La. State Univ.).

HEART DISEASE—DMSO plus hydrogen peroxide released oxygen to the heart muscle of small laboratory animals inflicted with a coronary artery closure. The combination seemed to protect the hearts from some damage (J. Finney et al., Baylor Univ. Med. Center, Dallas).

NERVE CONDUCTION—6 per cent DMSO slowed conduction of impulses along the isolated frog leg nerve (W. Mitchell Sams, Jr., Letterman General Hospital, San Francisco). DMSO exerted a reserpine-like tranquilizing effect, but it also lowered the convulsant threshold in animals—the effect could be overcome by the anti-convulsant alphaglucochloralose (AGC) (Monique C. Braude, Univ. of Md.).

TOXICITY—DMSO dosages ranging from weak to strong were injected into the veins of lightly anesthetized dogs with "remarkably few alterations" in heart-lung function, nerve reflexes and basic blood chemistry (Clare G. Peterson and Ralph D. Robertson, Univ. of Ore. Med. School).

ALLERGY—DMSO either prevented or greatly enhanced a type of allergic reaction known as the Schwartzman phenomenon. In this, an allergen is injected into the skin of the leg of a rabbit; when the same allergen later is injected into the vein there is a dramatic eruption at the previously prepared site on the leg. DMSO affects this, depending on how and when DMSO is administered. If 90 per cent DMSO is applied over the site where and when the allergen (a bacterial toxin) is injected into the skin, a later intravenous injection of the allergen results in a big and bloody reaction at the site of the first injection. If, however, the 90 per cent DMSO is applied to the skin at the time of the second toxin injection, it prevents the reaction completely. If a very small amount of 70 per cent DMSO is injected intravenously along with the toxin, death ensues within hours. While 70 per cent DMSO probably never would be injected intravenously, these experiments indicate that DMSO, concentrated, can be a two-edged weapon, capable of great good and possibly great harm in allergy (James R. Ward, Morgan L. Miller and Stanley Marcus, Univ. of Utah).

ENZYMES—DMSO dissolved every enzyme studied without irreversibly altering it. Inasmuch as enzymes often represent the chemical expression of specific genes, DMSO may help compensate for bad genes (D. H. Rammler, Syntex Research Institute, Palo Alto, Calif.). DMSO increases the activity of some enzymes (Carl Monder, Hospital for Joint Diseases, New York).

BLEEDING—DMSO, in different concentrations, seemed to control the mirror image dangers of bleeding and clotting. At under 1 per cent, DMSO speeds clotting; at 5 per cent or higher, it slows or prevents clotting (Herbert L. Davis et al., Univ. of Neb. College of Med.).

CELL SANITATION—DMSO has increased from ten- to a thousandfold the ability of cortisone and other chemicals to stabilize lysosomes, bags of the cells' scavenger enzymes (Gerald Weissmann et al., New York Univ.).

EYE DAMAGE—Dogs force-fed fifty times the human dose of DMSO five days a week for nine weeks developed changes in the lenses of their eyes. The changes cleared up, but not completely, when the DMSO was withdrawn. The same thing happened in rabbits and swine once or twice daily swabbed with high doses of DMSO for three months (Lionel F. Rubin, Univ. of Pa., and K. C. Barnett, Univ. of Cambridge). Rabbits fed about a hundred times the average human dose of DMSO for from seven to ten days developed lens changes which appear to be due to the loss of soluble proteins of the lens. The same dose applied to the rabbit skin was virtually without effect (Don C. Wood et al., Providence Hospital, Portland).

Dogs force-fed large quantities of DMSO for fourteen weeks and longer, developed a strange "lens with a double focus," much different than the change in refractive index caused by insulin, the sulfas, Diamox, aspirin-type compounds, ACTH and the miotics or as an aftermath to flu, rheumatism, tetany, jaundice, encephalitis, nephritis and TB (Kurt Eberhard Kleberger, Free Univ., Berlin).

A total of 108 patients with complaints involving 157 eyes were given 7.5–66 per cent DMSO topically for up to more than one year. Only one developed a lens opacity, which did not increase during nine additional months of DMSO therapy and was laid to causes other than therapy. The DMSO benefited patients with corneal edema and some, but not all, with eye inflammations (Dan M. Gordon, Cornell Med. School).

Thirty patients in Germany were treated for as long as eight weeks with DMSO in one series (and two hundred eighty others for various periods) without detectable ill effects on the eyes. "I think it should be mentioned that the topical dosages required to produce these (eye) changes in animals are astronomical in relation to the human dosage" (Gerhard Laudahn, Free Univ., Berlin, and Schering AG).

EPISIOTOMY PAIN—Topical application of DMSO for a few days following the severing of perineal tissues (to permit unimpeded birth and prevent the tears which sometimes result) reduced pain and edema but not enough to make the use of DMSO in this situation worthwhile (Irvin C. Arno et al., Albert Einstein Med. Center, Philadelphia).

CARCINOMA IN SITU—Barium-containing intra-uterine contraceptive devices often transform cervical smear cells into localized cancer or pre-malignant cells. DMSO with decadron alters the smears toward normal (J. Ernest Ayre and J. LeGuerrier, National Cytology Center, New York and Miami).

HORMONES—When DMSO was added, it increased the penetration of cortisol and testosterone through the skin 350 per cent (Howard I. Maibach, Univ. of Calif. Med. Center, San Francisco).

EAR, NOSE, THROAT—DMSO, alone and in combination with antibiotics (like tetracycline and erythromycin), wrought good to excellent results in such conditions as acute otitis media (but not chronic otitis media), nose or ear furuncles or inflamed pockets of pus, impetiginous eczema, tonsilitis and pharyngitis, aphthous stomatitis and malignant thyroid in the neuralgic type of head pain. DMSO widely applied to the forehead, neck and whole face sometimes provided sensational relief. Also benefited were temporomandibular neuralgia, hematoma (in which blood collects in a series of vestibules under the skin), cold sores and shingles (Hans Asen, Berlin).

ALCOHOL—In laboratory animals, DMSO, given beforehand, reduced deaths from lethal doses of alcohol; but DMSO increased the mortality when given after alcohol had taken effect. A pony of cognac will reduce the smell of DMSO (H. J. Mallach, Univ. of Tubingen, West Germany).

VETERINARY—DMSO often helps repair trauma effects in horses (M. D. Teigland, Florida Atlantic Univ.).

DMSO was of benefit in small animals with mammary engorgement, mastitis, post-surgical stasis, interdigital cysts and skin scurfing (Robert P. Knowles, Univ. of Miami).

It reduced considerably mortality from panleukopenia, a highly contagious blood disease of cats (Charles D. Dake of Ontario, Oregon).

When DMSO was painted on the open wounds of horses, it stimulated "fantastic" healthy granulation during the first few days; bacteriostatic properties were shown after a few days when badly contaminated wounds cleared up without pus formation, and a protective film formed over the wound surface. DMSO reduced excessive granulation to normal in one month (Francois Levesque, School of Veterinary Med., St. Hyacinthe, Canada).

POST-SURGICAL PAIN—Following open chest surgery for lung cancer, aortic aneurism, pulmonary tuberculosis, emphysema and hiatal hernia, the 12–15-inch thoracotomy incision was painted with 60–80 per cent DMSO every six hours. As compared with control patients, who received 10 per cent DMSO, the experimental subjects required only one half the usual amount of morphine and analgesics; and they coughed more easily, moved about better in and out of bed, had fewer complications (like ileus, nausea, vomiting and constipation). DMSO-treated patients did not develop pneumonia; and their post-operative course was less complicated and more rapid than that of the controls. Most subjects noted a moderate burning sensation during the first two or three applications; there was the odor, dryness and peeling; and DMSO was withdrawn from one patient who developed a localized rash (Dale S. Penrod et al., Pennsylvania Hospital, Philadelphia).

ACUTE MUSCULOSKELETAL CONDITIONS—A total of 187 patients with bursitis, tendinitis, sprains and strains in an uncontrolled series and ninety-two comparable others in a double-blind controlled series were treated with 60–90 per cent DMSO or, as a placebo, 10 per cent DMSO. A mathematical system of grading pain, tenderness, edema, limitation of motion, effectiveness and side effects was devised; and note was made of each patient's age, hair color, ethnic background, geographic origin and other variables. About 85 per cent of the DMSO-treated won excellent and good scores as compared with none of the placebo-treated; the pain scores for the DMSO-treated dropped from an initial 2.85 to 1.26 at one half hour, 0.45 at one hour, and 0.09 at seventy-two hours, whereas scores for the placebo-treated during the same periods were, respectively, 2.59, 2.55, 2.45 and 2.50. The investigator reported "dramatic and striking" results with DMSO (J. Harold Brown, Seattle).

Somewhat similar results in 1,025 cases of acute conditions were reported by German investigators. There were no side effects more serious than sensations of burning and itching (Heinz John and Gerhard Laudahn, Schering AG, Berlin).

CHRONIC CONDITIONS—Here, respectively, are the numbers of (A) cases, (B) partial remissions of symptoms, and (C) complete remissions of symptoms, and (D) failures reported after two or three months of DMSO treatment:

	(A)	(B)	(C)	(D)
OSTEOARTHRITIS	1641			
spine	896	253	539	104
hip	104	52	28	24
knee	497	202	215	80
small joints	144	46	69	29
RHEUMATOID ARTHRITIS	177	68	74	35
PERIPHERAL VASCULAR DISEASE	57	10	35	12

(John and Laudahn, Berlin)

MUSCULOSKELETAL, ACUTE AND CHRONIC—In 1,068 patients with acute and 848 with chronic disease, DMSO proved effective generally. Beneficial results were unpredictable, frequent and often dramatic, especially in acute conditions. Local irritation was troublesome. The potential for severe allergic reactions should be kept in mind (Christopher H. Demos et al., Squibb Institute for Medical Research, New Brunswick, N.J.).

ANESTHESIA—Tetracaine and other anesthetics dissolved in DMSO and applied to the skin of experimental animals produced prolonged anesthesia, and pain control for five days, without ill effect (Verne L. Brechner et al., Univ. of Calif. at Los Angeles).

ANTI-INFLAMMATION—DMSO, applied to the skin of 500 patients with diversified disorders, benefited 79 per cent. Acute conditions often cleared up completely, whereas long-standing chronic conditions tended to respond well only during treatment and for variable periods after it. Warming made DMSO more absorbent. When the pain was deep-seated—as in discogenic disease and radiculitis—ultrasonic therapy over the painted area enhanced absorption and hastened the response. Favorable responses (as measured by decreased swelling, increased mobility and other objective criteria, as well as pain relief) were achieved in these percentages: acute musculoskeletal injuries (whiplash, etc.) 81.1 per cent; osteo- and degenerative arthritis, 84.1 per cent (while under treatment); rheumatoid arthritis, 77.7 per cent; acute tendinitis and peritendinitis, 94 per cent; acute neuritis (from trauma, shingles, chilling, etc.), 88.2 per cent; acute synovitis and tenosynovitis, 88 per cent; discogenic disease, 50 per cent (poor responses in long-standing cases). DMSO treatment potentiated other drugs—insulin, digitalis, nitroglycerine—making it possible to lower the dosage (Arthur Steinberg, Albert Einstein Med. Center, Philadelphia).

GENITOURINARY—DMSO improved this number of patients: Peyronie's disease, 6 of 13; interstitial cystitis, 2 of 15; epididymitis, 7 of 12; herpes progenitalis, 2 of 5; polycystic kidney pain, 2 of 2; vague genital pain, 1 of 14 (Lester Persky and Bruce H. Stewart, Cleveland Clinic).

RHEUMATOID ARTHRITIS—Only one third of the twenty-one patients treated with DMSO alone or DMSO plus a steroid hormone showed good or excellent response. Many patients did not tolerate the preparation well (90 per cent DMSO in a total dose of 5 to 175 cc.). Skin wrinkling occurred after prolonged use. All side effects cleared up (Jack Zuckncr et al., St. Louis Univ.).

A carefully controlled study of 274 patients with rheumatoid arthritis sponsored by the Japanese Rheumatism Association showed that 50 per cent DMSO is considerably more effective and has fewer side effects than 90 per cent DMSO. Physical measurements and clinical tests were made periodically. About 50 or 60 per cent of the patients with moderate disease showed very good improvement on 50 per cent DMSO, as compared with about 40 per cent on 90 per cent DMSO. Good improvement was noted in 23 per cent and 16 per cent, respectively, of the advanced cases on 50 per cent and 90 per cent DMSO (Jun Matsumoto, Japanese Rheumatism Assn.).

HEADACHE—Of 154 patients with headache and/or neck pain and cranial neuralgia who applied 90 per cent DMSO to the pain areas several times a day, the results were excellent in 35, good in 60 and poor in 59. Some with two or more conditions, which might or might not be related, found that only one might clear up. Several reported improvement on placebos (Lester S. Blumenthal and Marvin Fuchs, George Washington Univ.).

SPORTS—Of 42 patients treated with DMSO for trauma, 23 were male athletes and 19 male or female non-athletes. Athletes and non-athletes responded in about the same percentages. The most important factor, generally, was time—whether the injury was old or fresh. About two thirds gave an excellent response, and almost all the rest a good response.

Among the many other conditions treated were: GOUT—Every one of the six patients had complete relief of pain within thirty minutes; DEGENERATIVE LUMBAR DISC—all but one of the 25 patients had a good or excellent temporary response; DEGENERATIVE CERVICAL DISC—10 of 16 patients had a good or excellent response; VARICOSE VEINS—21 of the 22 patients had a good or excellent response; ACUTE SINUSITIS—excellent response in six of the seven patients; THROMBOPHLEBITIS—all three with acute disease had an excellent response and the one with chronic a good result; STROKE —two patients showed unexpected improvement in damage from strokes that had occurred more than two years earlier (M. Marvin Paul, Toronto, Canada).

sports—Eight injured members of the Buffalo Bills football team who were treated with DMSO returned to duty in one half the usual time off for comparable injuries (L. Maxwell Lockie and Bernard M. Norcross, State Univ. of N.Y. at Buffalo).

scleroderma—This is a disease of unknown cause and no cure in which cell death creeps from fingertip ulcers and gangrenous toes throughout the body, calcifying subcutaneous tissues, paralyzing the digestive tract and attacking many organs. Of 42 patients treated with DMSO, 26 had an excellent or good response, with the disease not only arrested but actually clearing up in some of them. Three had returned to normal function and appearance and were able to withdraw—at least for a while—from therapy. DMSO caused a burning or itching sensation in many of the patients for a week or two. A few had nausea and loss of appetite until the dose was reduced. No side effect was considered serious. Among the symptoms which improved greatly or cleared up completely in many cases were gangrene of the feet, ulcers of the fingertips, decreased skin pigmentation, joint rigidity, tissue calcification, limited motion, pain and stiffness. Results of this sort "never have been observed with any other method of therapy" (Arthur L. Scherbel et al., Cleveland Clinic).

psoriasis—After a week or ten days of improvement, "the results were disastrous," and DMSO was withdrawn. Most of the 18 patients exhibited a sudden generalized psoriasis. This was due to "continuous application of DMSO in the concentrations used" (Marvin F. Engel, Brunswick, Ga.).

leprosy—Three groups of leprosy patients were treated with drugs dissolved in a DMSO skin wash, along with the oral antileprosy drug, Dapsone. Improvement was rapid and marked (Roy O. Yeats, Sopas Hospital, Wabag, New Guinea).

When Ruskin of the FDA had completed his talk, Arthur Scherbel of the Cleveland Clinic reminded him: "Doctor Ruskin, your group—Drs. Goddard, Sadusk and you among them—reported last week to the Fountain Committee that eye damage had occurred in 24 patients using DMSO. This report appeared in the newspapers. My patients, some of whom I was treating for scleroderma, came to me and said, 'Doctor Scherbel, you tell me there is no toxicity in DMSO, so far as eye damage is concerned, and the FDA says there is.' Dr. Ruskin, one of us is wrong. Would you please elaborate?"

Ruskin said that while there were a few reports of DMSO patients complaining of eye symptoms, no cause and effect relationship had been established. Ruskin didn't mention "the lady in Ireland."

This was perhaps the only time an official was called to account before an audience of scientists or physicians for the widely press-agented contention that DMSO had done serious damage to humans.

When they wheeled her into the emergency room that early February morning, the temperature outside the Rockford (Ill.) Memorial Hospital was 15° below zero, Fahrenheit, and her rectal temperature was 16.6° below normal. She had slipped on ice while stepping out of her car at midnight in front of her home, fallen to the ground, and for six hours lain there.

Dr. Forrest Riordan, former Assistant Professor of Surgery at Stanford University and now an orthopedic surgeon in Rockford, was called.

The patient, fifty-nine, was unresponsive to questioning; she moved frozen arms and legs restlessly, aimlessly. Heavy clothing had given some protection to most of the body, but both hands were blue, both knees a fluorescent red. Ice crystals could be felt in the knee bursae and in all the toes of the left foot and great toe of the right foot; and her feet, like her hands, were an ugly purple. The heart beat irregularly. There was no sensation in any of the discolored tissues.

Conventional treatment was begun in the intensive care unit. The patient, in a gown with protective leggings, was warmed gradually. The rectal temperature rose slowly to 85° at 9 A.M., to 95° at noon and 99.5° at 5 P.M. She was given intravenous fluid and, later, warm liquids, as well as one drug to relax her and another to steady the heartbeat.

The best of conventional therapies wasn't good enough. About six that evening, large blisters began to form on the toes, and the fingers began to turn black. Riordan applied 65 per cent DMSO from the wrists to the fingertips and from above the knees to the toes.

Since meeting Jacob at a Hand [Surgery] Society meeting in Chicago in 1964, Riordan had treated more than fifty patients with DMSO; and he had seen no side effects more serious than a rash or itch that subsided within an hour. He had witnessed the dramatic diminution of pain, often within minutes or a few hours of DMSO application, in a majority of patients with tendinitis, bursitis, bad bruises, sprains and strains, and even the unsightly injuries from automobile accidents and mechanical crushing.

He recalled that the English used DMSO for cold storage of living mammalian cells, young Charles Huggins' cooling of red cells and blood and Stanley Jacob's preservation of whole organs. Impelling too was the recent demonstration by the Virginia plastic surgeon J. E. Adamson that when a flap was produced surgically in the rat skin, DMSO improved the circulation to it and usually kept it alive. The question was: Would DMSO give new life to the lady's dying digits and restore the blood supply to her limbs?

Ten minutes after Riordan had swabbed DMSO on the patient's hands and lower legs, the treated areas reddened with the return of blood. The DMSO odor was on her breath, showing that the drug was permeating the woman's system.

On the second day, blisters had popped out on all the frozen areas, and that evening she regained consciousness.

The most cheering development came on the third day: sensation began returning to some of the toes, and later the tips of the long fingers began to have feeling again. By Day 7, she was able to flex these joints.

For an entire month, the patient was sloshed, swabbed and dabbed with DMSO. Almost one gallon of it was used, but side effects amounted only to an occasional rash, a bit of burning or itching (the cause for elation as numbness gave way), the typical

DMSO odor, and sloughing of the thawed skin. During the month the parameters of health returned to normal—body temperature, white blood cell count, sedimentation rate and other blood measurements. By Day 14, it was clear that all tissues were viable; and on Day 17 sensation at last returned to the knees, and only a few scabs showed where the blisters had been. The only other drugs prescribed were vitamins C, A and E.

The patient said that the accident and/or treatment had made the skin on her hands smoother and softer than it had been in twenty years, hair grew and it was rich and darker than before the accident, and her nails lost their earlier tendency to split or crack. By the end of the first year, cold and her first cigarette of the day made her long fingers turn white—a sign that circulation there wasn't entirely normal.

Riordan concluded that the drug should be applied within twelve hours of freezing and that twenty-four hours may mark the critical point for reversing damage to the involved blood vessels.

Frostbite is a common—and frequently a severe—occurrence, oftenest among traffic accident or immersion victims, or drunks. About 55,000 American soldiers in World War II and 7,000 in the Korean War were treated for cold injuries.

Don Wood produced laboratory proof of the usefulness of DMSO in frostbite. He shaved the ears of New Zealand rabbits, dipped one ear of each animal into an alcohol-solid carbon dioxide bath at −42° C., and then treated each rabbit with gauze pads dampened with 1) warm water, 2) 90 per cent DMSO, or 3) 68.4 per cent DMSO.

Groups (1) and (2) received no benefit from the treatment (warm water and 90 per cent DMSO, respectively); the frozen portions blackened in gangrene and fell off. Frozen tissues treated with 68.4 per cent DMSO, on the other hand, survived in many cases in a completely healthy state, and, generally, there was less tissue necrosis, edema and scarring.

When the animals' thighs were subjected to extreme cold, they responded as the ears had.

The most surprising results of all, however, came when DMSO was used to *prevent* frostbite damage. Tissues painted with either 90 per cent or 68.4 per cent DMSO remained undamaged in cold that brought gangrene and amputation to unprepared tissues.

Morris Green boarded Cloud Nine and returned from his triumphal tour of the West. He was a happy man.

Maddock had made a first-class presentation at the American Association for Cancer Research meeting in Denver. She couldn't miss; because, as was the custom at Sidney Farber's scientific citadel, the data had been put together meticulously, the text was modest, the conclusions scrupulously reasonable.

In Portland, Green had presented the same slides and the same material at a special seminar for the faculty. Even the members who had favored firing Jacob were well behaved.

The visit to Portland went so well, in fact, that Green relaxed in a jovial mood with the science writers who covered his lecture. He told Marge Davenport of the *Oregon Journal*: "DMSO is the agent that can get there fastest with the mostest. It is logical that it should now be tested on humans in connection with anticancer drugs." To Ann Sullivan of the *Oregonian* he said: "It is hoped there will be a release of DMSO by the governmental authorities to permit carefully controlled therapy trials with human beings." Both writers emphasized his statements that DMSO offered nothing at present for cancer patients. Like most science writers, they were careful to protect sources from their own indiscretions and from the cannibals haunting the scientific jungle.

When Green returned to Boston, he sent an account of his mission to Farber. He appended to it the text of his lecture and perhaps with a small proud flourish, the newspaper coverage of his visit.

In all this world no man was more determined to cure cancer than was Sidney Farber, M.D., Sc.D. (Hon.), the most famous in a family of distinguished physicians, Chairman of the Division of Laboratories and Research, the Children's Medical Hospital; Professor of Pathology, Harvard Medical School at the Children's Hospital; Director of Research, Children's Cancer Research Foundation; Member of the National Advisory Cancer Council; past President of the American Association of Pathologists and Bacteriologists, the Society for Pediatric Research, and the Worcester Foundation for Experimental Biology; Fellow of the American Academy of Arts and Sciences; member of the Leukemia Committee and Legislative Committee of the American Cancer Society; winner of numerous awards and honors, including the Lasker Prize, and frequently mentioned as candidate for the Nobel prize for Medicine.

He stood tall among the few giants who have made measurable contributions toward understanding cancer—Huggins, Hertz, Duran-Reynals, Haddow. He introduced antifolics which seem to be curing a childhood leukemia and a few solid tumors, like choriocarcinoma, and combinations of agents which cure a common cancer of the kidney. He employed, guided and inspired many productive researchers; and he instilled in them a strong sense of right and wrong and a rigid adherence to the protocols of science and medicine.

Children's Hospital is a monument to Farber's medical skill, scholarship and political sagacity. This is where great scientists and physicians from the far parts of the world come to discuss their programs and their progress, to study, to think, and to work for a while. This is where ideas are graduated from tests on cultured cells, to experimental animals and, if they get over that hurdle, to patients usually considered terminal. It is where Farber on appeals from physicians in many large and small centers, freely dispensed his counsel over the phone, where Farber has sweet-talked and wheedled key politicians into supporting the gargantuan growth of the federal cancer control program.

No distance was too great, no day too long for his unrelenting pace. It was as though time was running out on him. Sidney Farber was saved by great surgery from death by cancer of the colon many years ago; and specialists still prodded his scarred old heart to perform the heroic tasks he demanded of it.

Some who had worked for him, or with him, and who at one time considered themselves his friends, complained that Farber had sacrificed them to his stern sense of discipline. They contended that Sidney Farber had one responsibility, one desire, one passion, one love above all others—his mission in a world created for his destiny—to prevent any child from dying of cancer.

One can only speculate on the emotions that bubbled up on this busy day when Farber received Morris Green's report. With congressional committees to be begged for billions for the nation's research, with a welter of reports on matters within his own establishment to be read, with lectures and speeches to prepare for professional and public gatherings, acutely aware of the thin lines he must walk to favor this friend and to keep that enemy at bay and the delicate balance of humility and glory on which his "image" hung and, in the back of his mind, conscious of the to-do about dangerous DMSO, he read Green's glowing account and the clippings.

And he hit the ceiling.

He dictated a note firing Green.

"I have just instructed Dr. Maddock that you are not to be permitted into her department, or any of her laboratories, and that any work that you have been carrying on will be stopped at once," Farber wrote.

He added, "There are other aspects of this Oregon lecture which you gave without permission which I will take up with you personally next week at which time I will discuss with you your future plans. You do not have my permission to carry on any work in the Children's Cancer Research Foundation concerned with cancer."

Green became a casualty due to a ricochet in the war on DMSO. Others received a direct hit.

Call him Dr. X. He has had too much publicity—dished up by the FDA in its blacklisting procedure and reported prominently

116

and without question in public and professional media. The coverage did not constitute journalism's finest hour. Nor Dr. X's. Nor the FDA's.

The FDA charged that Dr. X had "falsified" his records in several ways: in reporting twenty-four weeks of testing DMSO on prisoner volunteers, whereas the prison records showed only sixteen weeks, and in the number of prisoners. Without knowing the charge, without counsel, or trial by judge and jury, Dr. X and all scientists associated with him had their names stricken forthwith from the list of those approved by the FDA for testing new experimental drugs.

Dr. X admitted inaccuracies in his data but contended that the errors were inadvertent and did not influence the final conclusions that the drug was safe. As a full professor at a leading Eastern university and president of three busy commercial laboratories specializing in drug testing, there had been too much detail for one man and a small staff to handle properly.

Dr. X was fully punished for any careless errors he had made. He had been caught by the FDA, tried (in absentia) by the FDA, convicted (in absentia) by the FDA, and given an unusual, and what some might consider, cruel punishment by the FDA—forty lashes in the press.

The way it was handled: FDA Deputy Commissioner Winton Rankin on July 19, 1966, sent out a letter to thirty-odd pharmaceutical companies stating that Dr. X had "failed to comply with the conditions applicable to the use of investigational drugs"; and he advised them to recall drugs then under his investigation. The FDA used a popular government device, the "news leak," and for reasons hard to understand, the press treated this shoddy story as privileged as though it had come from the Supreme Court or the Congressional Record.

In "reluctantly" confirming the Dr. X scandal, Rankin made it clear that, with all the damage done, Dr. X had been apprised of his misdeeds, and he could come now to the FDA and show where the bureau had been in error.

117

As a supposed finale to this innovation in dispensing justice, the FDA reinstated Dr. X after he had spent one month in the press-produced purgatory. On August 19, 1966, Rankin wrote to the drug companies that Dr. X and his associates "have instituted a number of significant changes in their procedures which make it possible for us to now regard [Dr. X] and the investigators associated with the three named corporations eligible to receive investigational drugs for clinical testing."

The quality of this mercy was thrice blessed—it blessed Dr. X et al. who could now face the world ready to find new happiness; it blessed the FDA and its press agents who had established a new and simple system of justice; and DMSO was dead, the FDA had killed it. Again.

Jacob, at the New York Academy symposium, received a message that Goddard would see him the next day in Washington.

I asked Jacob to note what transpired. This is his report:

I met with Dr. Goddard at 5:00 P.M. on the 17th of March, 1966. After a few pleasantries I sat down.

Dr. Goddard looked at me sternly and tapped his hand on the desk, saying, "Dr. Jacob, there are two very serious matters I have to discuss with you. The first is you have violated the hell out of these regulations. We gave you permission to treat a couple of hundred patients, and before that circus was over 50,000 patients were treated. I just don't know what to do about all of these violations. We have never seen anything like it. One of the things that bothers me, however, is that I can't find a motive. We know you didn't make any money from your activities.

"The second serious point is your accusation that my inspectors went into your personal correspondence files without permission. That isn't the story they told me."

I then related the story of the inspection. His answer was, "That's 180 degrees off the story my inspectors told me."

I said, "Dr. Goddard, did you look over all the material that was photocopied?" He said, "Yes, with the exception of 40 or 45 sheets of paper, everything seems relevant."

119

My answer was, "Do you think that there would be anything that was not relevant if I had given them permission?"

Dr. Goddard shook his head and said, "I just don't know what to do about you, Dr. Jacob. Your violations were terrible."

I had the feeling that Dr. Goddard was saying to me, you forget about the correspondence and I'll forget about the violations, although these words were not actually spoken.

There were strange noises on the telephones. With an army of FDA agents assigned to the DMSO patrol and, reportedly, more agents borrowed from the FBI for this purpose, Jacob and Rosenbaum felt they were under surveillance.

One day, Jacob said, "You know, Ed, until now I had never experienced the sensation of fear."

"Yes," Rosenbaum said.

"Now I know," Jacob went on. "For the first time in my life I know fear. I'm afraid for my family and myself. I'm afraid for doctors and scientists. And I'm more afraid for our country. I can't believe these things are happening in the United States."

Rosenbaum exploded: "Stan, everyone is advising us that the best thing we can do—and you in particular—is to lie low. When the FDA attacks in the press, don't reply; don't antagonize anyone."

Jacob said with rare impatience: "I *have* been keeping quiet. For one entire month, I have not answered the FDA. It doesn't work. More and more, they are slandering me and threatening in the press to prosecute me.

"The Jews in Germany remained quiet; they took the advice: Go along—everything will work out."

Rosenbaum too decided to fight.

When things were blackest, Jacob took comfort from the support shown him by his colleagues in the Department of Surgery, by Dean Baird, by many others, like Assistant Dean Joe Adams, Dr. William Krippaehne, Dr. Clare Peterson, Public Information Chief Ken Niehans, Bill Zimmerman, head of the business office,

Norm David, Chief of the Department of Pharmacology, and Dr. Joe Matarazzo, Head of the Department of Psychology, among them. Elsewhere, too, educators and scientists of stature and integrity were declining to compromise with the FDA.

The strongest support of all came from patients.

When the FDA banned the use of DMSO, those who had found in the drug surcease from sickness and pain protested. Most wrote to their Congressmen, some to the President or the Vice-President, others to the public through letters to newspaper editors. And some, hopefully, fervently, asked the FDA to change its course. Protests came from all parts of the United States.

Here are excerpts from a few of the letters in Dr. Jacob's possession:

I am a victim of arthritis. For many years I had not known what it meant to be free of pain. I experienced that wonderful feeling when I was treated with DMSO and improved greatly in my ability to move about with normal freedom. I cannot but believe that FDA has usurped power which rightly should be in the hands of medical researchers. It not only deprives victims of disease from blessed relief but it retards the work of dedicated researchers, and our country inevitably will lag behind other countries. [By a medical writer]

During my career as a medical specialist and medical officer for my country, I have seen many "miracle" drugs—penicillin, streptomycin, para-amino-salicylic acid and isoniazid. Also promazine and chlorpromazine. None of these had the immediate and spectacular results shown by DMSO. Nor did any have the future potential as a solvent and vehicle for other drugs. My personal experience began in 1964 when I read about DMSO in the local newspaper. I had had multiple bursitis since 1942 when I became so disabled in my right shoulder I could not use a bronchoscope or thoroscope. I had tingling, numbness and blanching of the fingers so bad I could not hold a fishing rod. Fearing I might have Raynaud's disease, I went to the Mayo Clinic. I had had multiple punctures, novocain, cortisone injections, diathermy, ultrasound and all forms of physical therapy with only temporary benefit. I had to support my elbow with pillows in the car and arrange the pillows to permit the "floating" of my shoulder during sleep.

Finally in 1964, when the pain became unbearable, I wrote to Dr. Jacob. Dr. Edward Rosenbaum treated me with DMSO. I took all the tests first. Then 15 minutes after DMSO, I noticed I could hang my arm without pain. Then I began to move my arm in all directions—for the first time in at least two years. I was free of pain until October, 1967—for more than three years—when pain recurred in my shoulder. I had used DMSO on burns, and there was no blistering, and no trauma, with prompt relief of pain and swelling. One application over the sinus region completely relieved a headache my assistant had had for three weeks.

We have potent drugs for the cure or control of most cases of tuberculosis; but kanamycin causes neurotoxicity and loss of hearing, viomycin and ethionamid liver toxicity and gastroenteritis, and myambutal occasional reversible blindness. Had these potent drugs been given full treatment by the FDA, as is given now to DMSO, patients with resistant TB bacilli would have to languish in hospitals for years.

I hope my comments both as a patient and physician may help give DMSO the trial it deserves for the sake of the suffering patient. [I.L.C., M.D., F.A.C.P.]

Dr. Goddard found it much easier to abdicate than do anything constructive about the [DMSO] matter—leaving the battle to the many who have been helped by DMSO, and not a single case reporting any ill, or side, effects worth noticing. Would you feel comfortable seeing *your* mother suffering the constant pain of arthritis with no other recourse except to become a dope addict just to enable her to tolerate the pain at all?

That is exactly the category I fitted into until DMSO bailed me out of that hell on earth. [Mrs. H.D.]

My brother Bob was unable to walk and was bedridden when he read about DMSO. He was being treated for hemophilia, but the doctor, not being sure of the drug and its use, would not prescribe it for him. Squibb referred Bob to an orthopedic man. Because Bob couldn't walk, he went to the doctor's office in a wheelchair.

After using DMSO daily for three weeks, he was on his feet again and able to go back to work.

My son, Bill, (also a bleeder) had joint pains and injuries, and I used it on him with marvelous results. We used it for my mother's bad neck burn, the hand which I smashed in a car door, and other matters, and with brief treatment with DMSO these healed miraculously.

My brother used the drug with excellent results until the FDA took it off the market. Perhaps the efforts of the Foundation will not go unheeded. [Mrs. M.H.]

I had a big toe operated on a dozen times that hurt so badly, constantly, I could hardly live with it. The doctor was trying DMSO experimentally but was not too sold on it, but he agreed to try it. He tried it for a week, but because I could not see that it helped much, we quit. A couple of days later, I suddenly realized that for the first time in months—or years—my toe did not hurt. Never since using DMSO have I had the pain in my operated toe again.

Now I have had spinal surgery four times, and there is nothing more can be done. But the intractable pain is driving me almost crazy. I'd like to try DMSO on my low back area. [B.J.M.]

I suffered a disarming attack of bursitis of my right shoulder during a field trip. I drove home with one arm, precariously and with the vibration of my car inducing unbelievable pain.

A friend, Dr. Norman David of the U. of O. Medical School referred me to Dr. Jacob, while my right arm had to be completely immobile by securing my elbow to my hip. Within 20 minutes after the first application of DMSO, a few inches of lateral movement was possible; applications at four-hour intervals permitted 90 per cent recovery on the second day and 100 per cent on the third day.

My experience is a relative inconvenience by comparison to hundreds who have suffered miseries far greater and obtained relief. [C.O.I.]

Early in 1964 my doctors treated my head with DMSO. The treatments, ten in all, healed the severe head pains which I had endured for more than nine years. Up to this time I had been given many drugs and treatments with no relief at all. [G.M.]

At 46, I was a deformed arthritic mass of pain from a childhood injury which shortened my left leg by healing with a short bend. Physicians thought I had been born with one leg shorter than the other; and this caused a severe curvature of the spine and, with age, arthritis.

Two hours after my first DMSO treatment, I felt a buzzing in my knee and my leg straightened—after 34 years. I then had treatments on my back. My spine is still curved, but nothing like it was. I am straight, my hips and shoulders lateral, not forward with an enlarged hip, and the lump of muscle doesn't show. I no longer have osteoarthritis in my knee and, at 51, I can drive a car long distances and teach a class in college. Before DMSO, I couldn't walk a block or ride 10 minutes in a car.

When I think of all the arthritics—including my mother—and when I think of my sitting at the New York Academy of Sciences Conference on DMSO and seeing the vastly successful indications (medical, industrial, agricultural) presented there, I can't believe what has happened to this drug.

FDA did not attend that conference to find the truth. They were, and still are, hoping for error, so they can justify the silly position they were scared into by the thalidomide crisis.

Please do all you can to see that your committee is aware of the importance of your bill to the health and welfare not only of your own people but to the peoples of the world who rely on you. [Mrs. P.H.J., writer-editor, member of the N. Y. Academy of Sciences]

During the eight months I have been testing DMSO, 1) I have been able to walk and drive a car (I had been consigned to a wheelchair by doctors at the University of Michigan Medical Center; 2) my terrible swallowing problem, due to a calcified esophagus, has improved although I still eat baby food meats; 3) I still have nine fingers left, free so far from amputation. I'm fighting for a change in drug evaluation to give thousands of other people a future of some promise. [J.D.]

I am severely handicapped with a progressive ossificating myositis.

It affects the muscles like arthritis affects the joints. The muscles become solid and the joints adamant.

My shoulders, elbows, right wrist, back, knees, and ankles are completely adamant. I have a little motion left in my fingers, left wrist and hips. My care depends on someone else's help 'cause my legs and arms are completely rigid.

My doctor, who I had for the twenty years of my ailment, has tried everything known in his specialized field of arthritis and rheumatism. In 1964, he sent me to Dr. Stanley Jacob to try DMSO. I used DMSO until the FDA put a halt to humans using it. That was one year since I was deprived of using the only medication that has helped my condition.

With DMSO my ailment was arrested and my nodes made smaller. I suffered less pain.

I have wrote the FDA, Dr. J. Goddard, about my case asking them to please release to my doctor some DMSO. Since the ban my ailment has progressed to a much more distressing condition than in 1964 before I started using DMSO. They have made no attempt to try and help my case. [K.L.W.]

I am the victim of a rare chronic systemic virus infection, which is not recognized by a majority of the medical profession. In 1965, I had an acute attack of encephalitis, hepatitis, and asthmatic bronchitis so severe that mental and speech coherence were impaired and I scarcely hoped to live through the night. The internist who had accepted me three months earlier gave me prednisone, which resulted in immediate improvement. But before the course was completed, serious symptoms of encephalitis recurred. I felt I had nothing to lose, as the next attack would almost certainly be fatal.

I tried DMSO strictly on my own responsibility. Results were truly dramatic. All symptoms diminished, and after an absence of six weeks I returned to work. Laboratory tests showed equally dramatic chemical improvement in liver and white cell count.

When I returned to work, the FDA halted all clinical testing of DMSO as eye lesions had appeared in laboratory animals given massive doses for six weeks or more. Being unwilling to sign false statements to obtain DMSO ostensibly for laboratory use, my condition deteriorated. Appeals to the FDA—whether directly, or through the federal agency where I am employed, or through members of the Senate and House, were of no avail. After much searching I was able to procure some DMSO in a nearby country. But when I had only two months of this supply left, I could obtain no more.

To preserve my life, I was forced to become either an expatriate or a smuggler. Since I could not earn a living abroad, I was compelled to adopt the latter course. It cost me a fortune.

I have been a law-abiding citizen, having been charged with nothing more serious than about six traffic violations during 40 years of driving. Because of the unconstitutional actions of the FDA, I have been forced to violate valid and necessary Federal laws in order to preserve my life. I believe this constitutes a very serious infringement of my constitutional rights, and, as such, is a matter of concern to the ACLU.

Since it is almost hopeless for an individual of modest means to challenge a Federal bureau in the courts, I respectfully request legal aid from the ACLU:

1) To seek an injunction barring FDA from search and seizure and other interference with *my* existing supply and medical use of DMSO;

2) To bar FDA, Customs, or the Department of Justice from prosecuting me for violations to protect my life;

3) To permit me to purchase DMSO to control my disease, subject only to a licensed physician.

Thousands of patients with crippling diseases and with diseases of progressive deterioration, ending with 100% assurance of mortality, are denied lifesaving DMSO by bureaucratic inertia and prejudice on the part of the FDA. [A.B.C.]

I attribute *all* of my success to DMSO for not having to go through with the amputation of my right leg. I was told by several professional men I would not be able to stand the pain otherwise, and they were right. The pain was so excruciating, so severe that I bounced my head on the wall. I had to crawl instead of walking, and I took 15 to 20 painkiller pills a day.

With all this in mind, I was brought in a wheelchair to see Dr. Jacob. Thank God for that day. From that day on, I began using less and less pills, until there was nothing but DMSO. I walked, did my own shopping, my own housework.

For two long years this wonderful drug has been kept away. How many people have lost their limbs during this time? Tying the hands of Dr. Jacob in my estimation is an unforgiveable sin. Please, please let DMSO come back to us. [E.M.F.]

No lovelorn swain, no homesick soldier in a faraway jungle, no starving student looked forward to the postman more avidly than Stanley Jacob did. Through his mail he learned which battles he was winning, which losing, and how went the war on its multitude of fronts—with the FDA, in Congress, with the plethoric pathology that beset his patients, with organized scientists, individual doctors, with creditors, with admirers and critics.

The mailman endowed Jacob with the gift of total ubiquity— the vicarious power of being everywhere at all times.

Fortunately, Jacob was a fast reader. A glance gave him the contents of a page. He was rapid at dictation. Usually he could absorb his incoming mail and dictate a few dozen letters in a couple of hours.

Jacob's day was long and busy. It often began in the middle of the night with emergency surgery. Four mornings a week, between about eight-thirty and noon, he was either operating or in the clinic seeing patients scheduled for surgery. He himself seldom saw more than twenty of the fifty or sixty patients reporting to the surgical clinic; but in the clinic he instructed medical students in diagnosis and treatment. The twenty-eight beds in the state-operated medical school surgical ward were occupied by patients beyond the expertise of most surgeons or the procedure called for equipment unavailable elsewhere. The University of Oregon Medical School long had been famous for its surgical teams; its students saw many rare surgical problems and performances that they never again came upon in their careers as surgeons.

Jacob's day was crammed with administrative duties, animal research, visits with surgical patients, a course on one day for each of six weeks for twelve to fifteen seniors on the fundamentals of operating room behavior—aseptic conditions, tying, handling surgical instruments. Using one dog for no more than one single surgical procedure (after which it is "put to sleep"), he had the students insert a tracheotomy tube into the neck, explore the interior of the belly, suture a nerve in the neck, take out part of the thyroid, hook up sections of the digestive tract, and, in the final session, divide the great aorta leading from the heart and sew it together again.

Two nights a week, Jacob treated fifteen or twenty patients with DMSO. At this rate, thirty or forty a week, he had given more than four thousand treatments with DMSO by 1972.

Some of the most bizarre conditions were seen at his DMSO clinic. Many patients became his friends and corresponded with him for years. He seemed to bleed a little with those he couldn't help and die a little with those who came to the end of the road.

There was, for instance, a case of myositis ossificans generalis, which is so rare that some voluminous medical references fail to list it. Furthermore, they might just as well ignore it; there is nothing the patient can do except die. Slowly.

A man in his thirties had had the disease for twenty years. In 1964 Jacob started him on DMSO, and after a few months (of topical application) he had improved. When they had started out, a good deal of his body had calcified—he couldn't move any of his joints; he couldn't lie, or sit other than rigidly; he couldn't bend his neck or move his fingers. His knees, his hips, his ankles—all were rigid. But he could open and close his mouth; so he could eat, and, for the time, survive.

"We concentrated on his shoulders," Jacob told me, "because I felt that if we could get a little motion in the upper part of his body, it would make him less of a vegetable. After a couple of months, he did recover some shoulder motion. Then, gradually, some of the calcified soft tissue lumps became smaller and smaller.

"When the FDA halted studies in November 1965, the young

man had regained much use of his fingers; he wrote, literally, hundreds of letters—to the FDA, to Congressmen, and to the President. The FDA sent him stereotyped letters. The President, who receives a lot of touching personal appeals every day, overlooked this one.

"In time, special permission was given to the doctor to resume treatment. Naturally, the patient would have to submit to frequent, time-consuming and financially debilitating tests."

Other diseases were equally baffling but a good deal more common. One was Lou Gehrig disease, or amyotrophic lateral sclerosis; Jacob treated a neighbor of mine with DMSO and wrought some instant, overnight and slightly delayed wonders of therapy. But from my own knowledge, he was never permitted to pursue this line of investigation; my neighbor's physician forbade DMSO.

One patient with multiple sclerosis was about twenty-nine when she came from another state to Oregon for treatment for the virulent disease. Not only was she paralyzed, but she also suffered from kidney failure to the point that she was trying to induce those operating the University of Washington dialysis program to save her. At this time one could be saved for perhaps nine who had to be rejected for help on the artificial kidney machine.

Jacob started the MS patient on a high dose of DMSO, two ounces a day—but dabbed on. Then, with great daring, he and his associates gave her the DMSO orally—a stiff dose in tomato juice or orange juice.

"Her improvement was dramatic—as dramatic as any benefit I have ever seen," Jacob told me. "Within a week her renal problem seemed to come under control. Then—after a few more weeks—she walked again.

"Now, six years after her first DMSO treatment, she still has wobbly knees. But she walks. She drives her car. She takes care of her two children and her husband. But she is going downhill. I wish we could help her again, but we just don't seem able to. Despite this, however, I am not convinced that DMSO alone is useful in multiple sclerosis."

Marge Davenport of the *Oregon Journal* engineered what she hoped would be a practical solution to Jacob's problems with the FDA. She persuaded Congressman Robert Duncan of Oregon to bring together in Washington representatives of both sides—the FDA and DMSO advocates—and let them thresh out the issues in the presence of the press.

On October 5, 1966, the entire cast gathered around the conference table. Duncan was referee. On the side of the government were Goddard, Hodges, Ruskin, Dr. Milton Silverman (representing HEW Secretary Dr. John Gardner) and FDA press agents. On the scientists' side were Jacob, Dr. Lester Blumenthal of George Washington University, who had found DMSO effective against headache and neuralgia, Dr. Arthur Scherbel of the Cleveland Clinic, who had used DMSO as an effective treatment for heretofore untreatable scleroderma, Dr. Marcus Mason of the Mason Research Institute, Worcester, Massachusetts, who had reported DMSO remarkably non-toxic in animals, Dr. Dan Gordon of Cornell Medical School, who attested to DMSO's efficacy in some eye diseases and to its lack of toxicity to the human eye, and Dr. J. Harold Brown of Seattle, and the dean of American pharmacologists, Dr. Chauncey Leake.

The press was not admitted during the discussion.

Goddard and Hodges opened the session and dominated it. They dwelt at length on the supposed toxicity of DMSO.

Jacob told me later, "No one at the meeting spoke up. We wanted the FDA to save face and get off the hook gracefully."

Jacob said that when he started talking about DMSO's use against conditions which could not be treated well by other means, Goddard cut him off with the observation that he was a highly prejudiced observer.

Jacob gave me this account: "I suggested that some of the differences between the scientific community and the FDA on DMSO could be resolved by the National Academy of Sciences. Dr. Goddard replied that the suggestion was very similar to one advanced by Dr. Andrew Ivy during the Krebiozen matter."

The press was called into Duncan's office and once again, Goddard took over. "He answered all the questions," Jacob told me. "There wasn't much opportunity for any of the investigators to say a word."

"What did you do?" I asked.

"I talked to the reporters outside the office—after Goddard had gone," he said.

Because crusades, for good ends and bad, cannot be conducted successfully in Washington without the aid of a professional and costly lobby, DMSO's legislative support proved weak and ineffective.

The Oregon delegation—especially Senator Mark Hatfield and Rep. Wendell Wyatt, both Republicans, and Rep. Edith Green, Democrat—worked heroically for DMSO. They had arranged for the Library of Congress to reproduce and translate any DMSO scientific papers published abroad.

Wyatt conducted a series of rebukes to the FDA on the floor of the house. The orations appeared in the Congressional Record under the standing headline, "DMSO, the Persecuted Drug." When Goddard's agents were most active, Wyatt said:

"Thousands of people in this country are needlessly suffering because of the FDA's arbitrary holdup of clinical testing of

DMSO. The holdup is pure futile arrogance on the part of a Government agency.

"In thousands of documented cases, suffering has been alleviated, pain reduced, and symptoms have disappeared; but in not one single case had a serious side effect been discovered. Restrictions on its use make companies and doctors alike shrink from even filing an application to test this drug. FDA actions have been so harsh, in fact, that drug companies refuse to make DMSO available in medically acceptable grade. The FDA has been accused of bludgeoning the medical community into submission . . . of forcing submission to its orders by blacklisting investigators, threatening scientists with unwarranted court action, conviction by press release and, in general, using questionable methods to control the actions of the medical profession."

Thanks to the Oregon delegation's intervention, the Library of Congress at this time began supplying Jacob with reprints and English translations of DMSO papers in foreign journals.

The first two were by groups of Italian dermatologists. Here are my abstracts of them:

A cream containing an antibiotic (neomycin sulfate) and a cortisone-type hormone (9-a-fluoroprednisolone 21 acetate) was divided into two batches: Batch A, containing DMSO, and Batch B without DMSO.

Batch A was applied to eczema and dermatitis sores on the right sides of 24 patients, and Batch B to sores on left sides of the same 24 patients. Treatments ran from 2 to 20 days. Based on the rapidity and completeness of healing, results were graded excellent, good, or incomplete.

Batch A—containing DMSO—was superior to Batch B in 16 cases, inferior in 2, and the same in 6. [Prof. F. Serri, University of Pavia, *Minerva Dermatologica* 41 (1966)]

Combinations of DMSO, the cortisone-type hormone, triamcinolone acetonide, carbopol, and propylene glycol were applied to 90 patients with various skin conditions.

Prof. Bella found that the combination, with considerable consistency, proved far more effective against most of the skin conditions than the cortisone-type hormone alone. Various combinations often yielded excellent results in such conditions as eczema and psoriasis.

With DMSO serving as a vehicle to transport it into the deep skin layers, triamcinolone acetonide doses could be cut to 10 per cent of normal; and except for the typical DMSO odor, taste, and brief burning sensation, the drug was well tolerated, and without ill effects. [S. Bella of the Dermatological Hospital Institute of S. Maria e S. Gallicano, Rome; *Minerva Dermatologica* 41 (1966)]

Jacob read the papers with interest—and also with a touch of sadness. He wondered whether he would continue to receive reprints from abroad. Or had the FDA quenched research with DMSO throughout the entire scientific world?

The third international symposium, November 8 and 9, 1966, in the elegant old Palais Pallavicini in Vienna, was sponsored by the University of Vienna Medical School and financed by the German drug house Schering AG. It attracted 150 scientists from twelve countries.

Leake, as keynoter, said, "Rarely has a new drug come so quickly to the judgment of the members of the health professions, with so much verifiable data, from so many parts of the world, both experimentally and clinically, as to safety and efficacy.

"Fortunately, members of the health professions throughout the world are not all bound by the bureaucratic regulations and judgments of the U. S. Food and Drug Administration."

It was strange hearing this statesman of science in this hall and this city, which less than a generation ago had been occupied by one of the bloodiest regimes in all history, now apologize for regimentation in America.

As at the Berlin and New York symposia, scientists said they had failed to induce eye damage with DMSO in any animal species close to the human, and they could find no evidence of eye troubles attributable to DMSO in any patient.

They reported that under certain conditions DMSO would a) overcome edema and other effects of trauma; b) carry the anticoagulant heparin through the skin and into the bloodstream; c) sharpen tests for kidney and liver function; d) damage the bore of arteries and veins when injected into them in concentrations higher than 30 per cent; e) reduce body water and both sodium and potassium (90 per cent DMSO, topically, increased urine volume ten-fold); f) with compound 48/80, DMSO prevented the calcifying effect of metal salts like lead acetate, and when DMSO was applied to the animal skin prior to giving 48/80 it preserved mast cells—treasure-houses of anti-coagulant and anti-inflammation chemicals—in injured tissues; g) given to mice ten days before infection, DMSO prevented typhus; h) it tended to solubilize collagen, a possible anti-aging effect; i) and in very preliminary observations, DMSO seemed to make resistant tubercle bacilli vulnerable to drugs—subsequent studies cast doubt on this effect, however.

In human studies—many controlled—DMSO reportedly a) relieved pain and sped healing; b) cleared up headaches associated with cervical disease or shoulder-hand syndrome; c) benefited 77 per cent of patients with rheumatoid arthritis and 84 per cent with osteoarthritis; d) transported the anti-cancer drug 5-FU and antiviral 5-IDU through the skin; e) helped scleroderma patients in controlling contractures, calcinosis and skin manifestations; f) offset some injurious effects of cobalt radiation therapy; g) proved superior to all other therapy for winter and other sports injuries; h) controlled many kinds of pain, including that associated with blood clots; and i) cleared up benign skin growths of the eyelids and neck by dissolving the oily fats which caused them.

Scores of scientists had confirmed the majority of the claims Jacob had made; and some had added new and original claims of therapeutic values. Jacob felt vindicated at the end of the symposium. The distinguished scientists clustered around him, shook his hand, congratulated him for what some called a classical contribution to science and medicine.

The entire assemblage seemed in a happy mood. All except one —Bob Herschler, who said not one word to Jacob or Rosenbaum or Leake. He stood aside alone and in silence.

At the Vienna conference it became known that Germany, without fanfare, was restoring DMSO to the drugstore shelves. There were more than adequate safeguards. It was a prescription drug, limited to topical application for specific ailments. It could not be applied for more than fourteen days at a time to anyone and under no circumstances to pregnant women. Germany became the first of a gradually growing number of countries who became disenchanted with the United States Food and Drug Administration and who quietly made DMSO available to doctors and their patients.

The three classical approaches to the development of therapies are: 1) empiricism—the trial-and-error testing, with or without a rationale, in hope of effecting a cure; 2) serendipity—the chance, or fortuitous, discovery by the alert and prepared mind; and 3) the biochemical, or orthomolecular, in which a specific compound is used to correct a known chemical defect.

Jacob adopted all three approaches.

Once he had satisfied himself that DMSO was extremely safe and remarkably effective against an assortment of conditions, he experimented boldly and empirically against many other diseases.

And when a chance observation suggested that DMSO might prove useful against new diseases, he lost no time testing it. Like the legendary Three Princes of Serendip, who sought one thing and found another of even greater value, Jacob treated one disease and discovered that DMSO tended to cure another in the same patient.

The story of Nate Amato illustrates serendipity.

Back in 1916 Nate and some other kids had built a fire over a handful of dynamite caps they had found in an empty house. They lit dry sticks and scattered to wait for the explosion. When nothing happened, one of the older boys said, "Nate, go over and see what's the matter." As Nate bent over the fire, the caps went off, and the dirt and rocks crashed against his face. The left eye had to come out. And the right eye gradually deteriorated. Three years after the accident Nate dropped out of school because he couldn't read or even see the blackboard; and eventually he couldn't distinguish light from dark. He bought a filling station and, even though blind, got along all right.

Nate heard that one of his customers, Dr. Jacob, was experimenting with some magic stuff called DMSO; and one day when Jacob stopped for gas, Nate asked, "You think DMSO might help this eye that I've got left but can't see out of?"

Nate had been blind for more than thirty years. Nevertheless, Jacob told him to bring a complete report from his eye doctor to the lab on Wednesday evening. Nate did and ever since then he has visited the lab on Wednesday nights—always first in line. He comes a little early, bringing Jacob a hamburger sandwich drowned in Tabasco sauce, because Jacob doesn't have time for dinner on the nights he sees DMSO patients.

Nate has not regained any vision; the only thing that's different since he started applying DMSO to his scalp and then by eyecup, first over the lid and then to the eye itself, is that he has a sensation of flashes. The intensity varies; the flashes are brighter on sunny days than on cloudy days.

One day Nate noticed a remarkable thing: running his fingers over his bald head, he detected traces of very fine hair growth—like peach fuzz, only maybe a little sparser. He felt that he knew the answer; Jacob had told him that one of the effects of DMSO was to dilate, to open up, the fine blood vessels in the skin, and it now was obvious to Nate that with a new nutrient supply, the follicles were producing hair where hair had not been growing for many years.

It was to be expected, of course, no one would credit the story of DMSO's growing hair on a bald head. Nevertheless, Jacob applied DMSO regularly—or prescribed it—to five more bald men.

Hair, of sorts, grew on all the bald heads—a fine fuzz that appears in the scalp areas where hair last grew and then spreads to other sites in inverse order of its disappearance during the balding process. Ed Rosenbaum was one of the five with some evidence of returning fuzz, but he still was not convinced that DMSO was responsible.

Nate once had a whiplash injury which his doctor felt triggered an arthritis attack; the x-rays showed degenerative arthritis in his right hip. "I began applying DMSO a year later," he said, "and I haven't had any trouble ever since." Nobody calls him cured, of course.

Amato is a down-to-earth, unemotional sort of fellow. Diagnostic x-rays confirm his arthritis story, and a series of snapshots show the growth of hair, very slowly, over several years.

He tells this story of his enlarged prostate:

> It could happen with age, I guess. I was having to get up a couple of times during the night. I was developing pressure in that area.
>
> Before this I was being treated by a doctor at the Portland Clinic; and I'd gotten to the point where the doctor suggested that I should have an operation for an enlarged prostate. I put it off and asked Dr. Jacob to see what he could do. My doctor told me to try it if I felt like it.
>
> Dr. Jacob tried DMSO with a series of prostate massages. The pressure disappeared. I no longer had to get up during the night; I sleep until six-thirty or seven-thirty in the morning without having to go to the lavatory. I have no discomfort whatever. That was sixteen or seventeen months ago. I still get treated occasionally. But that condition is under control.

Jacob told me that a physician in Texas some years earlier had reported injecting DMSO plus progesterone, the "pregnancy hormone," into enlarged prostates and that biopsies, examined under the microscope, indicated a return toward normal.

Vision never did return to Amato's eye.

Jacob took some satisfaction from the effects of DMSO on

137

Amato's bald head, arthritic spine and enlarged prostate. But he felt a keen sense of frustration that DMSO could do nothing for his blindness. The sensation of flashes that Nate reported, however, made it impossible for Jacob to abandon the idea that DMSO might help in some kinds of blindness.

Harry E. Palmer had spent most of his adult life in the field of public health. Up to the time of his retirement, he had been a lay psychologist for the state of Oregon.

Palmer and his wife had been diagnosed as having osteoarthritis. Mrs. Palmer's condition had become chronic. To open her hand with the locked finger, she had to reach around with the good hand and pry the bad one open. Harry had always been a little crippled as a result of old injuries; but it was only after he started laying tile in his retirement home down near the Oregon coast, that it really hit him.

"I got to the point where I could hardly walk up those thirty-five steps that led across the terrace from the street and up to the second floor bedrooms," he told me. "I came to know each one of those steps individually—as a challenge."

When Harry was on top of a twenty-five-foot ladder painting the house, his knees almost gave out. He stopped dabbing at the gable and climbed back to the ground—painfully, carefully.

Harry's mother had been one of the first patients treated in Jacob's lab six or seven years earlier; and ever since then, periodic treatments had kept the terrible pains in her knees under very good control. So Mr. and Mrs. Palmer asked Jacob to treat their arthritis.

"Dr. Jacob sat and talked with us for about an hour and a half, and then he accepted us for his arthritis program," Harry told me. "I just brushed the DMSO liberally around my knees and on my hands with a camel's hair brush. My wife dipped her hands in DMSO.

"The treatment was excellent for my wife's hands and fingers.

Now there's hardly any deformity at all. As for me, within three months I was able to run up and down those thirty-five steps.

"It is a new life for both of us."

During one conversation, Jacob said, "Harry, how would you like to try for a new head of hair—natural hair?"

Jacob showed Palmer some before (bald) heads in pictures and snapshots of the same heads, now not so bald, after several months and years of DMSO treatment.

"I didn't hesitate," Palmer said. "I signed right up."

"I now have fine hair on the back of my head almost an inch long; and it may be starting to come back in other areas too. However, it will take years for me to develop a decent head of hair."

Once again, serendipity intervened, and Harry Palmer's eyes became the beneficiary.

When he was ten years old Harry had roller-skated downhill and was hit by an automobile. He was unconscious for two days and not expected to live. When he was able to, he started reading a book, rubbed his left eye and screamed out, "Mother, I'm blind." That was when he realized the sight was gone completely from his right eye.

The ophthalmologists said nothing ever could be done for the right eye, and they predicted that Harry would lose the remaining sight in his left eye within six months. Thanks to the perseverance of one of them, however, some vision was preserved in the left eye. The right eye was sightless—dead; it wouldn't even focus.

"After I had used DMSO on my head for baldness for a few weeks, I began to have a strange new sensation back of my sightless right eye," Palmer told me. "I can't say it was pain, but it wasn't comfortable. It was sort of a dull ache.

"Oddly enough the left eye—that's the one that still had some sight left, not much but some—wasn't affected at all.

"Dr. Jacob had often advised us to tell him of anything unusual, so I told him about my right eye. He asked me if I'd be willing to go ahead with an experiment and bathe my eye directly in DMSO. I told him of course I would.

"We tried DMSO in various percentages. It caused quite a reaction. It stings for several minutes before it subsides, and tears run as when you get something in your eye. The eye is bloodshot for fifteen or twenty minutes, and the reaction lasts maybe a half-hour."

One day in Jacob's office, they blindfolded the left eye; and with only vision from his blind right eye, Palmer was able to describe objects that Jacob held at a distance. Then, faltering somewhat but without bumping into anything, he walked around a strange laboratory.

From that point on, Palmer's progress was fast and life was exciting. His pupils accommodated to light; his eyes focused; and then there was the supreme thrill—he could detect color (something he had not been able to do since before his accident) and name each shade correctly.

Jacob decided to test DMSO on an entire series of patients with "incurable" nerve blindness.

Late in May 1967, I carried my tape recorder into Goddard's big, shiny new office in the big, shiny new building, furnished in the modern manner of the fat and happy government of an affluent society. There were handsome trophies here and there—gifts from celebrated admirers in exotic areas of the globe.

My interview, with Goddard, assisted by an aide, Dr. Robert Hodges, ran for more than two hours and the transcript covered thirty-five pages of dialogue, single-spaced. It started off pleasantly. Goddard said, amiably enough, "You never saw two Irishmen who didn't want to get into a discussion, did you?"

I said, "It's usually in a saloon, though."

He said, "Sorry about that."

I pointed out that scientists at the New York and Vienna DMSO symposia were almost unanimous in citing the drug's fine therapeutic effects and minimal side effects.

"This is not our information," Goddard said. "I think we hear from different parts of the scientific community and I think this is quite natural. Advocates of a position often tend to go to meetings and present their experiences with a drug.

"Just last week a physician here was very enthusiastic about a limited use of DMSO. He found that by mixing the drug with a local anesthetic he gets a much better anesthesia than he does with any other single agent. It enables him to perform certain surgical procedures that otherwise are very difficult and have an element of danger connected with them.

"But the point of interest was that he brought with him some toxicity studies that I hadn't seen heretofore. These were carried out on the West Coast in association with a university medical center. As I recall, six of the ten developed leukopenia with administrations of small amounts of DMSO. Now, leukopenia—we view decreases in the white cell count as serious, and these were in the order of magnitude of three thousand white cell decreases from the normal.

"The striking thing was that there were eight patients out of ten who showed drops. [To Hodges] How did that go? It was six of eight ultimately, wasn't it?"

Hodges said he didn't know; he wasn't present. He did say that the white counts returned to normal, and the scientist was halfway through a rerun when all experiments with DMSO were terminated. Hodges said he "assumed" that at this point it was three of the patients who again were showing leukopenia.

Goddard said that, although he was familiar with the general DMSO literature, "Who was aware of this? I submit, some of these kinds of reports haven't received the study and attention of the general community."

Within the first few minutes of our interview, in his impressive presentation, Goddard was inconsistent himself at a time when scientists committing comparable mistakes were wrongly threatened with criminal action and disgrace.

I wondered too at his acceptance of a sketchy white cell depression as a critical situation. Some might wonder whether the agent might not be worth testing against leukemia, which is characterized by too many white cells.

Neither Goddard nor Hodges could identify the scientist immediately. I came across him later and found that his story varied considerably from Goddard's, as we shall see.

Despite the vagueness of his facts, Goddard expressed enthusiasm for the toxicity he felt he had discovered. He said it was "fascinating—one would not have expected this kind of dose response. Intriguing! And the consistency with which it occurred!"

"Now, a lot of comments have been made about the eye problem," Goddard said. "How do we really know it's only in animals? As I recall, there have been only seventy-one individuals in whom follow-up eye examinations have been carried out—out of the many thousands of people who received the drug when it was being distributed so widely."

Again, Goddard's figures were at variance with others'. (More than 600 such cases had been reported at this time.) I asked him, "How many patients do you have eye reports on who have been taking aspirin?"

"With any drug, when there is a suggestion of a problem based on animal studies or clinical observations, we insist on additional studies in humans," he replied. "Now, I know of no animal studies citing difficulties with aspirin."

I reminded Goddard that aspirin's toxicity was real and had been widely reported.

With considerable cutting, the interview covered such points as:

GODDARD Every drug has its toxicity. Now, I think we've demonstrated time and time again with our new drug approvals during this past year that we're not sitting here to block good therapeutic agents from coming into the marketplace. Rather, we're here because there has been a job placed upon us through the scientific community and Congress.

I You've frightened investigators to death. One gave up on DMSO in his blood-freezing technique. He told others—not me—it was just too risky to use.

142

GODDARD Let's put a little of the responsibility on the people who acted in an irresponsible fashion. We had a tough job of taking the action, that's true. But by the same token, those who acted so irresponsibly caused this action to take place.

Now, there's no question that we now have enough information that we are evaluating and looking at to consider changes in the policy statement which would broaden the testing.

I think we're very close to coming up with a policy statement that will open up studies.

I Are there as many as fifty patients in the United States being treated with DMSO?

GODDARD Yes, there are.

I Where are they?

HODGES I can tell you. They're throughout the country. There are about sixteen investigators and I should imagine about fifty or sixty patients receiving the drug. These have all been followed very carefully. We're doing now what the investigators should have done three years ago. We are completing Phase Two, the evaluations of late safety, Phase One and Two, in human beings.

I You are aware of the letters from patients and their families stating that the patients are in enormous pain which cannot be controlled by any means other than DMSO. What is your attitude, Dr. Goddard, to children who must live in pain?

GODDARD Well, first of all, in all cases where the physician wrote us, we have evaluated each of these on an individual basis and then we took action accordingly.

HODGES Dr. Goddard delegated to me the deciding of whether or not an application should be approved in conditions where there is pain or the patients have to be on narcotics, where they have life-threatening conditions. Scleroderma is one we are all well aware of. If they have severe pain from rheumatoid arthritis that was crippling and are not responding to anything else, I would not refuse approval. In fact, I don't know of any cases offhand where I have refused approval. I can't name one.

143

I   If I said I had seen letters to the effect that you had either refused or made availability of the drug impossible—

GODDARD   Well, let's clearly define what you mean by making availability impossible. We will approve an individual's request and then he must obtain a sponsor.

HODGES   Yes, and it's still a study, even though they're treating a patient who is seriously ill. It must be carried out with full regard for the patient's safety. They have to do these eye studies and blood studies to show there are no effects on the marrow, liver and kidneys. There is nothing to stop any practitioner who is sufficiently motivated. These studies cannot be done by the average general practitioner.

I   If it's so simple, how do you account for so little use of DMSO in patients who need it?

GODDARD   First of all, many physicians aren't willing to carry out the studies required for Phase Two.

I   Could another reason be that the physician then becomes subject to visits, let's call them, by plainclothes policemen, armed—

GODDARD   I take exception to that. Our investigators are not armed. We request our FDA field staff, our inspectors, to visit scientists and obtain certain data on their usage of DMSO—and their accountability for the amounts they'd received and used. This was done after a congressional hearing.

I   What happens if the researchers decline to make the records available?

GODDARD   Then we have to go to court and ask for a subpoena.

I   Have they entered laboratories in the absence of investigators and gotten records?

GODDARD   They have never obtained records without permission of the investigator. In one instance the investigator couldn't be there during the entire visit, because he was greatly involved in shipping DMSO to persons around the country. He told his secretary to provide them with the records. The university in that

144

same instance also instructed the person involved to turn the records over to the FDA inspectors.

This has been looked into very carefully, because some allegations have been made that we have acted improperly. We're prepared to defend our inspectors' activities on this.

I   Have your inspectors entered laboratorics and physicians' offices without an appointment?

GODDARD   Not without permission.

I   What kind of permission?

GODDARD   Go to the person in charge and identify themselves—tell them the purpose of their visit and what they are seeking.

I   But they don't make prior appointments?

GODDARD   They try to.

I   They do try to?

HODGES   Not always.

GODDARD   They try to in many instances.

I   If someone quoted your agents as saying they were required to enter the physician's office without prior notice, would that someone be lying?

GODDARD   That would depend on the circumstances.

HODGES   Many of our inspectors go to the physician's office and say, "Here we are, and this is what we want to see."

GODDARD   But they identify themselves—and do not enter without permission.

I   Despite its [DMSO's] willy-nilly use, uncontrolled, on eighty thousand or more people, so far as is known it has been without a single serious side effect.

GODDARD   Not so far as is known. Who followed up on thc people? Who checked up on them? There has been reported at least one instance of anaphylactic death.

145

I   The lady in Ireland?

GODDARD   Yes.

I   She was taking several things. Are you familiar with the circumstances?

GODDARD   Yes.

I   And you still say that?

GODDARD   I say there is one case reported. Now look, this is why facts are needed.

I mentioned that I had heard from Dr. X, who had been blacklisted, libeled and slandered, before being reinstated.

Goddard said Dr. X "has proper recourse if he feels he's been damaged in a fashion that's not appropriate. He can take this to the courts and sue us and sue me. If he's willing to do that, I'm perfectly willing to go to court on it. There's no problem there."

I had been denied data on DMSO from his office on the grounds that the facts were "confidential." Goddard commented: "That's quite appropriate—part of the policies we operate under. And I must say these are known to Congress too."

Regarding the quality of FDA scientists, Goddard said there were some good ones, but "like any organization, we have all gradations."

I told him he had been criticized as a czar of medicine with only one or two years in private practice and, reputedly, "without a very distinguished record."

"Nobody ever came to evaluate the quality of medical care I dispensed in my practice," he said. "How can they make that evaluation?"

I told him the critics were speculating.

"That I wasn't successful?" he responded with considerable spirit. "That I couldn't make a go of it? Let me tell you that last year for the first time, my salary equaled what I was making when I quit the practice of medicine in 1951.

"I submit to being in practice for fourteen months [in Kalida, Ohio] and grossing over twenty thousand dollars a year. You're not unsuccessful when you're charging two dollars for an office call (including the medication) and twenty-five for an obstetrical case (prenatal, delivery and the medication). It was a very busy practice, if that's a measure of success. In fact, that was the reason I quit. I didn't want to devote eighteen to twenty hours a day and have to practice in a fashion that I didn't think measured up to my own standards. I don't think that seeing forty to fifty patients a day and delivering up to a hundred babies in the last twelve months was exactly a good brand of medicine."

As for his being a czar of medicine: "I think that charge is ridiculous on the face of it. We don't have the ability to handle the practice of medicine in this agency."

I asked whether Goddard made mistakes, and he said, "You can't be an activist type of organization and not make mistakes." I asked what kind of mistakes he had made in the last year, and he said he had made some poor placements within the FDA. He added that he would have handled the vitamin controversy differently. (In this case, the FDA was caught attributing to the National Research Council the old FDA fetish against vitamins—proposing to compel the labeling of vitamin bottles with an announcement that people got enough vitamins normally from the food they ate. The council made the FDA recant.)

Apropos of Goddard's admitted mistakes, I asked whether he thought it fair to prosecute Dr. X and others. Did it seem that for him and the FDA to err was human but scientists' bookkeeping mistakes were criminal offenses?

"To err is human," Goddard said. "But to submit false data, which is not an error, is not human."

Reputable investigators had presented data at the Vienna meeting on more than ten thousand cases treated with DMSO which the FDA was ignoring; the cancer findings alone were urgent enough to be checked, I suggested.

"With cancer," Goddard said, "during this period, we stood

147

prepared to receive and approve any protocol on the treatment of cancer. Did we receive any?"

"No," said Hodges.

I asked, "Doesn't it make you wonder why you didn't?"

There was no direct answer.

Goddard complained that the DMSO story appeared first in the public press.

I pointed out that he and the FDA were having a terrible time keeping things from the press, that somehow news did get out of his office into the papers and on radio and TV.

He confessed that news leaked out of the FDA. "There are leaks everywhere," he explained.

Goddard insisted that the FDA was merciful: instead of taking an erring scientist or doctor into court, it merely blacklisted him.

"A lot depends on the nature of the individual case," he said. "We make that assessment, and we always meet with the investigator, give him an opportunity to come in and show us where we've been wrong. So far this has been a workable system."

Was it fair to listen to the man's story *after* destroying him? I said, "Well, it's been workable from your point of view. But take the investigator whose reputation is shot, his career is over. No one again will trust him after a trial in the press initiated by the FDA."

Goddard heatedly denied that the FDA initiated a "kangaroo court in the press."

It was Hodges who finally explained the practice:

"Well, how the present situation arose is when we first found these [drug testers], we wrote to the sponsors of the investigation, notifying them that they were no longer acceptable investigators. This is picked up in the drug trade news that such and such a person is no longer an acceptable investigator, whereupon the ordinary lay press came down here and wanted full details on the first case. It was very much garbled; and since then we have made a practice of issuing a short press release after the notice has gone to the drug firm."

I asked Goddard if he deplored the fact that his news on blacklisting got into the hands of the press.

"We recognize the reality that it does," he said. "And so once the letters have had time to reach the sponsors, we simply put out a press release that says the investigations related to this investigator—the sponsoring firms have been notified."

I raised the question of whether Goddard and some of the press had not committed libel.

"We stand to be sued," he said. "Any investigator who thinks he's been treated unfairly has recourse to the courts. He can go and hire a lawyer and get us in court."

I said I thought that in view of Goddard's own "human mistakes" and his getting into the press so much, he'd have understanding, if not sympathy, for Stanley Jacob.

"I have a sympathy with the scientific community in this whole issue," he said. "But we're not talking about actions taken on the publicity. We're talking about actions related to the record keeping, the patient information, the studies that were supposed to be carried out."

I brought up the charge that the number of new drugs in the United States had fallen to an all-time low and that the FDA was responsible.

"I think that's pure baloney," Goddard said. "New drug applications started to decline in 1956 and have been going down ever since." He said that neither the FDA nor the Kefauver Amendments was responsible.

Goddard said that scientific knowledge, on which drug development is based, is cyclical. "I happen to be very confident that within about five years we're going to see the development of a great many more important products than we have today."

A friend had told me he had little hope of overcoming the FDA's formidable barriers to the general availability of two potent immune hormones he had isolated—at least for a long time.

"The question of length of time isn't what we're discussing," Goddard said. "We're talking about whether a product gets on the market or not."

How about making available drugs to relieve pain and cure sickness in people now ill?

"We're interested in truncating the time too," he said, "but part of that truncation is the responsibility of the investigators. Just what happened in DMSO can slow up the availability of the product to the people in pain, and that's the function of the investigators doing good studies."

Goddard's tension could be measured in two ways: by the number of cigarettes he smoked—and on this occasion, he sometimes had two burning simultaneously—and by the beat of his fingers on the long conference table. The tape shows that at this point the beat was a fortissimo.

Would Goddard guess as to when DMSO might be marketable if efficacy for scleroderma and a few other conditions were proved —or it turned out to be an effective pain-killer?

"Within six months after the new drug application has been submitted, a judgment will be made by the FDA," he said.

That was back in the spring of 1967.

My interview with Goddard left a disquieting sense that many—perhaps most—of the officials' statements were in error.

Goddard reported with a straight face that there was substantial criticism of DMSO at the New York Academy and Vienna symposia. I covered both meetings. His word was hearsay and wrong.

When he complained of the paucity of eye examinations during DMSO treatment, he ignored 310 patients under John and Laudahn, Scherbel's 47, Jacob's and Rosenbaum's 25, D. Hoffmann's 25, A. H. Kutcher's 84, Gordon's 108.

His intimation that a sizable number of patients were under treatment at the Cleveland Clinic was not so. Scherbel had been forced to discontinue his studies.

Scherbel explained the situation in a note to me: "I believe it would be most difficult, if not dangerous, for any clinical investigator to again start studies with DMSO while the FDA remains biased and emotionally prejudiced against the drug." He said, "On the surface, FDA regulations appear acceptable to all concerned. It is readily apparent that large numbers of patients in a special study program cannot be seen at four-week intervals for prolonged or indefinite periods. The expense of laboratory studies as well as the expense of medical personnel make the study prohibitive.

Grants are not available because of lack of interest (by drug companies and granting agencies) in these studies."

Scherbel said neither the patients nor the clinic could spare the money; and the families couldn't spend the time to bring the patients in and home again. He pointed out that in the event of abnormal findings (chemical or otherwise)—which would be inevitable—the additional studies demanded by the FDA would prove impossible. Eye examinations required half of a patient's day, and the law prohibited driving with the degree of dilatation that would result.

Among the points that struck me as especially noteworthy were Goddard's defense of his police and their methods, his unsmiling reference to the poor, dead "lady in Ireland," his denial of enormous influence over the professions, his exculpation of the FDA in the personal and professional reputations it had destroyed, his rape of the—it must be said willing and consenting—press, and his readiness to pit the power of the government against aggrieved citizens in costly and time-consuming litigation. His minimizing of the disastrous trend in drug development and his optimistic prediction that things would soon pick up.

Even Goddard's boast that he grossed $20,000 a year (which ordinarily would mean about $12,000 net) as a small-town busy doctor for a total of fourteen months could be interpreted in many ways.

The week after my Goddard interview and a few months after the FDA had reinstated Dr. X and given his story a happy ending, I received a note from Dr. X.

"I am the person who was so badly mauled by the FDA last year," he wrote. "Although there may be no connection, the National Institutes of Health have just disapproved two major grants upon which I was strongly depending." He said he would have to get rid of his research personnel and abandon much of his experimental work on aging, if funds were not forthcoming.

I referred him to the American Cancer Society officer who headed up the research grant section, and I added:

Last week, I had the pleasure of an informal chat with Dr. Goddard. Among the many topics in this candid conversation was the FDA's use of libel to punish some scientists and threats of it to keep others in line.

Your name in particular came up; and I told him then, as I told others at the time of FDA's attack on you, that it is a pity you did not sue him and his agency for libel. You now seem to be reaping the fruits of your timidity.

While Dr. Goddard did not agree with my attitude on this and many other matters, he did say he would welcome the opportunity to go into court to present his defense against the charges. I earnestly hope he has this opportunity.

Dr. X may have been correct in not suing. He was fifty years old, at the peak of his productive career, and with quite a few obligations to his family. The suit could leave him penniless, in debt and further scandalized.

Dr. X would stand little chance against officials of the FDA, their own police, the agents of other federal departments, a staff of government attorneys and incalculable resources available at the expense of the taxpayers.

Shortly thereafter, Dr. X put it this way:

My survival instinct has prevented me from taking a public stand in my own defense. You must appreciate the fact that the FDA has complete power to exterminate me by the simple process of making me ineligible [to do research with experimental drugs].

Their actions can easily lead to my annihilation in the university. The academic community and industry are so completely intimidated that one cannot look for any leadership to counteract some of the punitive actions of the FDA. I find that my name has been permanently blackened in the minds of some persons and some agencies.

I see no way of winning a battle with the FDA, and I have decided not to be a dead hero, or even a useless one. I am very pessimistic concerning the future status of medical research unless a mood arises to combat overzealous bureaucratic authority.

I am bewildered, resentful, and without too much cheer concerning my future status. Perhaps I prefer the illusion that such things really cannot happen in America and that sooner or later sense and decency will return.

Incidentally, I am usually regarded as a person who has more than average courage. In this case, my policy is surely not the courageous one, but I hope it is the more rational.

Goddard and his associates had promised to send me evidence of DMSO's serious toxicity in humans. At this writing many years later, I still ask the FDA occasionally for the references.

One document, purporting to represent some evidence, was a bibliography of twenty-three scientific papers. I was familiar with most of them, and I searched and was able to dig up all the rest. Not one of them carried any data indicating human toxicity beyond the slight and fleeting odor, occasional transient itching and sensation of heat, a splotch of rash that might last a few hours, or pustules that were gone overnight. When there was any doubt at all, I wrote to the authors. Every single one denied that he had reported or knew of instances of lethal or serious DMSO toxicity in man.

The bibliography sent me by the FDA did include hostile papers—a half-dozen or so. They attacked Jacob mainly for the newspaper accounts and they showed a pretty sour interpretation of DMSO treatment data, or, in some cases, inferior results. Patient improvement or deterioration under treatment often lay in the eyes of the clinical beholder. Improvement in, let us say, one third of arthritic patients could stir enthusiasm in one investigator or bitter criticism in another.

Charles Lebo, M.D., of the University of California Medical Center in San Francisco, it turned out, was the investigator who had induced what Goddard had called a dangerous leukopenia in humans. He did not share Goddard's interpretation, or his "facts" or his alarm.

Lebo's technique called for instilling five drops of 50 per cent or 60 per cent DMSO three times a day into the right ears of convict volunteers for more than two months. Lebo established the complete safety of DMSO when given in this manner. The results suggested that an anesthetic might be mixed with DMSO and instilled into the ear to permit the safe and relatively painless surgical puncture of the eardrum, a procedure which patients otherwise find excruciating. Encouraged by Lebo's and similar experiments, others have utilized this procedure with considerable success.

Lebo's periodic examinations of the subjects—multiple blood counts, complete physicals (including ear, eye, nose, throat, etc.), bacteriology, and blood and fluid chemistry—showed only odor was a side effect, and the convicts did not find it objectionable. As for the leukopenia, Lebo reported that, everything considered, "the validity of this finding is open to question." Since it never before or since has been reproduced, Goddard's reference to it as "intriguing" and "consistent" hardly seems warranted.

Denny L. Tuffanelli, M.D., a University of California dermatologist, had an article in the *Archives of Dermatology*, Volume 93, June 1966, which led off with: "In view of enthusiastic reports concerning the use of DMSO in scleroderma, a clinical trial with this agent was carried out. Twenty-four patients with systemic scleroderma were treated with local applications of DMSO. Under the conditions of this study, no improvement of any of the parameters studied was noted."

Tuffanelli said he would have terminated the study, except that "a continually increasing number of patients referred to our clinic sought DMSO therapy because of the enthusiastic 'lay' press reports."

It is redundant to say that the scleroderma patients were in a bad way. Gangrene was beginning to eat away at their fingers and toes; and if Tuffanelli knew of a better treatment for the disease, he didn't mention it. Progressive amputation of the extremities is conventional medicine's answer to this phase of scleroderma; but there are uglier and more baffling aspects, for which amputation (of the esophagus, for instance) is hardly the answer.

Tuffanelli reported giving his patients the complete physicals and other tests required by the FDA during their treatment, which averaged 4.2 months. Mathematically, in nineteen patients with a total of thirty-one fingertip and toe ulcerations, five in the treated patients healed and three new ones developed during the study; in untreated patients the score was six and four.

"Unfortunately," Tuffanelli complained, "the lay press had led afflicted persons to expect DMSO to be a miracle drug."

Some patients and doctors reported better luck with DMSO.

One such patient, Mrs. John Barlet lives in New Castle, Pennsylvania, and works hard in a ceramics plant. She spends a good deal of time trying to contact other scleroderma patients—she says there are 50,000 of them in the United States—to give them a little booklet on their disease. When I received a copy of her letter, she had been in touch with eighty-nine.

After being treated "for everything but scleroderma," she went to the Cleveland Clinic. She told Dr. Arthur Scherbel there how the pain had started in her shoulders about two years earlier, then went to her hands, which took on a grape juice color when cold and swelled and ached until eventually ulcers began to form on her fingertips.

"My face was swollen with pulled eyes and tight, glassy-looking skin," Mrs. Barlet wrote. "I had much trouble breathing, and there were pains in my chest quite often. Large calcium lumps which crippled two fingers on the left hand and one on the right hand formed. I would get tired easily, couldn't lift or carry anything, couldn't open a tiny lid on a jar. The skin always looked suntanned, and tiny broken veins showed up like blemishes. I had always been a very active person with no illness whatsoever."

Scherbel diagnosed it as systemic scleroderma with secondary Raynaud's phenomenon. He put Mrs. Barlet on Marplan, which is used against angina and depression, the anti-cancer agent methotrexate—and DMSO. She has been on this for years.

"I have been one of the fortunate few to be treated with DMSO, by a doctor researcher, with fantastic results!!!" Mrs. Barlet wrote. "This has turned my condition in reverse, with freedom of movement in my hands and joints; it has softened the skin; the swellings have disappeared; the ulcers on the fingertips cleared, better breathing, the skin has returned to normal. I very seldom have pains, and I do not tire as easily. I certainly know what this drug can do!!!"

Mrs. Barlet began writing for fellow scleroderma sufferers when she was fifty-two years old and had had the disease for seven years, five of them on DMSO. "When it was reported that the National Academy of Sciences might spend 18 months studying DMSO," she protested, "we scleroderma patients are going to continue to deteriorate without the use of DMSO."

"We need and want DMSO now," she added. "When I think of how the many suffering people could be free of pain and crippling, and can't have it, I become very SAD. The drug is very cheap to process and is a poor man's drug, which is the greatest drawback of all. No one can make any money on it. It entered the servants door and was never accepted." She ended with: "I Remain Your Scleroderma Friend."

Leonard Marmor, M.D., and Barbara Walike, R.N., of the University of California at Los Angeles wrote in *California Medicine* of July 1966 how they treated fifty-three rheumatoid arthritis patients with DMSO.

Marmor and Walike began their article: "Dimethylsulfoxide (DMSO) since its public introduction in a news release from the University of Oregon in December 1963 has been the center of a great deal of publicity and numerous discussions and reports. Little has been reported in medical journals, although many readers of news reports seem to have concluded that DMSO has unlimited uses."

Of the fifty-three—all of whom had advanced (Grades III and

IV) disease—thirty-three received no benefit, twelve fair results (some temporary improvement up to six hours), and eight good (pronounced improvement up to twelve hours, including definite pain relief). This spelled failure in 63 per cent of the cases and success, of sorts, in only 37 per cent, little better than placebo effect.

The way Marmor and Walike put it: "The experience with DMSO therapy herein reported does not seem to bear out the tremendous publicity given the drug. Fewer than 40% of patients with rheumatoid arthritis in the present series had a good or fair result despite the fact that many may have been prejudiced toward the drug by the publicity in lay publications. (It is well known that 30% or more patients will experience a placebo effect from any medication given with therapeutic intent.)"

Sixty other patients—treated for osteoarthritis, bursitis, tenosynovitis, etc.—didn't do well either.

The UCLA patients suffered abundant but evidently brief side effects; only seventeen reported having none.

A laudatory article about Marmor's surgical technique in rheumatoid arthritis later appeared in the *Reader's Digest*.

Only one other report emphasized side effects. The investigator —patently hostile, not only in his reports but also on the Portland campus—retired into complete obscurity without publishing anything beyond his pre-preliminary observations, which were lacking in data.

Not one of the authors mentioned in the FDA's bibliography of twenty-three papers claimed to have the slightest evidence that DMSO had caused serious toxicity in humans. I asked them.

Typical of replies to my queries were:

From D. A. Willoughby, pathologist of St. Bartholomew's Hospital, London: "We failed to demonstrate anti-inflammatory activity and found, on the contrary that DMSO produced irritant activity. As far as we are concerned, DMSO is a useful compound for producing inflammation in experimental conditions. In this respect, we find DMSO a powerful and possibly dangerous irritant. This is not to say that under proper conditions it may not have some uses when used judiciously."

From F. Caujolle, Director of the Centre de Recherches sur les Toxicités, Toulouse, France: "You will note that all our results were obtained on animals and naturally cannot be transposed to man."

From George I. Malinin, Biomedical Research Institute, Rockville, Md.: "Toxicological properties of DMSO were not under investigation and consequently no claims were made that DMSO is toxic when used in pharmacological concentrations."

Tuffanelli wrote me: "We did not feel that DMSO was toxic as we used it, though there were a few cases of irritant dermatitis. However, its effectiveness was not impressive under the conditions of our studies."

There were differences of opinion and some contradictions in facts expressed by various scientists. P. Görög, Ph.D., of United Pharmaceutical Works, Budapest, Hungary, reported that in rat paw injuries DMSO had an anti-inflammatory effect. This was, in a sense, the opposite of what Willoughby had reported, possibly due to different subjects, different kinds of inflammation, different dosages, rebound phenomena or any of a dozen factors.

The FDA and its spokesmen damned and for many years suppressed DMSO because of its toxicity. What is DMSO's toxicity?

Stanley Jacob, Ed Rosenbaum and perhaps every other expert will agree that any drug can kill any person. If it is given in too high a dose, by an unwise route, in combination with certain other treatments, at the wrong time of a chemical or physical cycle, to an overly sensitive patient or one with organs unable to detoxify it, or to one too young or too old to metabolize it—the drug, any drug, can kill. And perhaps all, or almost all, of the commonly used drugs have contributed to human death at one time or another.

DMSO can kill. But there is no reasonable evidence that it has ever seriously harmed a person. Nevertheless, those who know DMSO best regard it as potentially lethal. It induces a histamine-release reaction occasionally, and if this were severe enough it would send a person into shock. In all the literature I have reviewed and all the authorites I have interviewed, I have not come across a case of DMSO-induced shock.

Animals have been killed with DMSO. They were killed deliberately and with difficulty. A group at the Mason Research Institute in Worcester, Mass., once analyzed the data from their own and fourteen other groups' experiments and found it takes a lot of DMSO to kill mice, rabbits, rats, guinea pigs, chickens, cats, dogs and monkeys. The drug was given to the animals by mouth, or total immersion to their necks, or by injection into or under the skin, and into the mucous membranes, veins, muscle, bladder, lymph ducts, belly cavity and eye. When enough DMSO was applied to or pumped into the animals for long enough, they became crippled and died. The initial harm in most cases was to the eyes— lens clouding and nearsightedness (not cataracts); next came liver damage and destruction of red blood cells. When rats were immersed up to their necks and sopped up 100 per cent DMSO, all of them died. But when concentrated DMSO was painted on their entire skins daily for as long as three months, the damage was minimal. And when mice and rats were completely immersed up to the ears in DMSO concentrations similar to those painted on the human skin—60 or 70 per cent—all survived repeated treatments.

The Worcester group—Emil R. Smith, Ph.D., Zareh Hadidian, Ph.D., and Marcus M. Mason, D.V.M.,—commented in their article in the September–October 1968 issue of *The Journal of Clinical Pharmacology* that any animal which survived immersion—a thorough dipping—for as long as twenty-four hours would not die of DMSO toxicity. Rats dipped three times a week for six months showed ulcerous dots on the belly and back skin and slight changes in the blood and liver. All effects were reversible.

Dogs and monkeys given whopping doses of DMSO, as much as 3.3 per cent of their body weight applied to their skin every week for six months, showed only one adverse effect—halitosis.

The Smith group established what is called the LD-50, or lethal dose 50 per cent, meaning the amount of DMSO necessary to kill one half the test animals. They concluded: "It is readily apparent from these LD-50 values, as indeed it has been apparent from all of the other studies discussed above, that DMSO possesses a very low systemic toxicity."

LD-50 by injections ranged as high as 0.8 per cent of body weight when given intravenously to mouse, rat, rabbit, dog and monkey. It was two or more times that for intraperitoneal and subcutaneous injection and about three times that—or 2.4 and 2.8 per cent respectively of the mouse and rat body weight when DMSO was taken by mouth. Rabbits, dogs and monkeys were able to take only 1.4, 1.0 and 0.4 per cent of their body weight of DMSO orally to have one half their number survive.

The local damage done by injections depended to considerable extent on the concentration of the DMSO—the higher, the more damage. Here again, in single doses, no matter how much DMSO was given or by what route, if the animal survived twenty-four hours, it was out of the woods—all signs and symptoms of toxicity would disappear, most of them within a week. Among the local symptoms usually seen was the typical inflammatory reaction and irritation of the injected area of the vein; a hemorrhagic, gelatinous and edematous lesion at the site of muscular or subcutaneous injections; local constriction of the vessels, followed by hemorrhage and necrosis, when 100 per cent DMSO was injected intradermally; a transient (three-to-twelve-hour) formation of exudate on injection of 25 per cent DMSO into the rat pleura, the sac encasing a lung.

A group from Toulouse, France, headed by Drs. F. M. E. and D. H. Caujolle, reported finding liver damage in animals which succumbed to very high doses of DMSO given orally over a period of days, or intravenously or intraperitoneally in doses amounting to as much as 1 per cent of the animal's weight. When dripped into a vein, or perfused, 50 per cent DMSO was used. "On the basis of these acute and chronic studies, in mice, rats, and dogs," the French group reported, "it appears that the acute toxicity of DMSO is not great; even relatively high doses of DMSO (in 50 per cent strength) are apparently well tolerated. However, these results by no means indicate that DMSO is nontoxic. The chronic toxicity studies, despite the short period during which the drug was administered, indicate that DMSO does have a toxic potential."

The Caujolle group injected 50 per cent DMSO into chicken

eggs after eighteen to twenty-four hours of incubation; and they established the LD-50, and the maximum non-fatal and the minimum always-fatal doses. "From these data," they reported, "it appears that the toxicity of DMSO toward the embryo is low." One in four chicks that survived the LD-50 showed malformations, mostly of the limbs but also of the eye, beak and other structures.

The Caujolles injected DMSO repeatedly into the bellies of newly pregnant mice and rats, and about 7 per cent of them bore offspring with malformed limbs and other defects. When the DMSO was given in low dose but regularly in drinking water to pregnant animals, the baby rats and mice were sound. The mammalian mothers tolerated toxic doses of DMSO well, but the fetuses did show the effects of DMSO—but only when relatively high and repeated doses were given.

Caujolle told me that—contrary to FDA insinuations—his findings did not imply that DMSO might deform human babies. This seems reasonable, because, for one thing, very few women are likely to be injected in the belly with DMSO during pregnancy. At least, not repeatedly. Or anyway, with enormous doses. And, especially, not during the earlier months, when nature's construction of various embryonic organs could be interfered with.

One other animal, the hamster, was sensitive to the teratogenic effects of DMSO.

Don Wood of Portland was among the first to investigate extensively the effects of DMSO on the functioning of organs and the metabolism of laboratory animals.

A quiet, amiable scholar with tremendous patience, Wood administered DMSO in various doses and by several routes and traced it to its ultimate excretion. He made not only an organ by organ check, but he also analyzed what the DMSO did in different cells and cell structures. He measured its influence in the synthesis, activity and breakdown of compounds in the blood, other fluids and many tissues.

Wood showed that even in the three species susceptible to eye

163

changes under massive doses of DMSO, the effects were by no means blinding. Working mainly on rabbits (dogs and swine were the other susceptible species), he discovered that large doses over long periods changed the lens so that the eye became more and more myopic—nearsighted or shortsighted. One group said subtle changes were noticeable in swine after ninety days of 90 per cent DMSO twice daily. Wood and his co-workers effected lens changes in rabbits in two or three weeks by giving them—by mouth and painted on the skin—DMSO doses amounting to 1 per cent of their body weight per day. He emphasized that DMSO does not cause cataracts.

Some reported that, to a degree, the lens changes were reversible, although no one was able to undo the damage completely.

Even ultra-high dosages failed to induce eye changes in other species, most significantly monkeys (only lethal and near-lethal doses induced lens changes).

Mason summed up: "It is of the utmost importance to point out that changes in [animal] lenses were consistently seen only when high doses were repeatedly used over an extended period. The routes used to elicit the changes were oral and dermal. It is also noteworthy that in none of the reports on eye changes was there mention of alteration in the visual acuity of the subject. Dogs never showed difficulty in running, jumping, or avoiding obstacles, despite a marked change in lens refraction."

Animal studies showed that if humans reacted as do the average in the most susceptible species, none of them closely related to the human, it might take a pound or two of DMSO a day to do damage. A pound or two of DMSO could last a sick, accident-prone, bruised, arthritic family for months.

The properties which make DMSO unique—especially its ability to dissolve other substances and transport them through the skin and into the bloodstream—pose a theoretical danger. Should a poison or an infectious material (like cyanide or viral DNA or RNA) contaminate DMSO applied to the patient's skin, what would happen? DMSO will inactivate and detoxify some harmful substances; but we will never know which until broad-scale research resumes.

It has been shown that rats injected in the belly with DMSO and given carbon tetrachloride by stomach tube, will suffer awesome liver damage—more than with tetrachloride alone. Few humans can be expected to take carbon tetrachloride by stomach tube while being injected in the belly with DMSO.

Periodically over the years, the FDA has announced that DMSO research will soon resume—or, indeed, that it already is under way. Few centers have the specialists and equipment needed. Consequently, there were very few such studies. When I called this to the attention of FDA officials, they explained, "Well, we can't force doctors to undertake the studies, can we?" Or, "We can't compel pharmaceutical houses to handle DMSO; if they're afraid of a visit from our inspectors, there's nothing we can do about it." Or, always, "We're only enforcing the law."

Looking back on it now—through the rearview mirror—the afternoon of May 19, 1967, may have been a turning point in the careers of Goddard and Jacob.

This was the day when the two men held, as Goddard had proposed it, a "doctor-to-doctor meeting," in the FDA office in Seattle. Jacob, his confidence in Goddard badly shaken after two confrontations with him, still believed the commissioner when he said legal matters would not be discussed but, if he wished, he might bring his attorney to the meeting. Jacob went alone. He was seeking vindication; the alternative could mean lengthy criminal litigation, scandal, professional unfrocking, prison—ruin.

Goddard probably was seeking his own vindication. At stake was the reputation of the FDA as a serious enforcement agency and justification for its police actions. One friendly agent had told Jacob, "It would take a major catastrophe—like a botulinus epidemic—for the FDA to remove any of its men now working on the DMSO matter."

FDA agents had entered many of Crown's warehouses in Camas and smashed bottles of DMSO. One of the Syntex officers, a German refugee, had said FDA operations at Syntex were reminiscent of Nazi Gestapo tactics. A Pfizer officer had been grilled repeatedly by FDA agents; a principal point of interest was: Had there been

166

collusion among the drug houses to hide DMSO toxicity or make unwarranted therapeutic claims?

Rosenbaum said that, so far as he could learn, only scientists who had found clinical value in DMSO had been harassed by the FDA.

Jacob was a problem. When he caught the FDA agents copying his personal correspondence, he had them thrown off the campus. After being muffled at a press conference, Jacob went to the reporters and offered his side of the story. Now he was proclaiming that his rights as a physician superseded the powers of a government agency.

Goddard smiled and stuck out his hand when Jacob came into the Seattle office of the FDA. Jacob described the event in a memorandum to Norm Kobin, his lawyer:

"Dr. Goddard said that he had been wrestling with the question of my 'violations' of the Food and Drug Administration regulations for a long time. He mentioned that he had considered three possible alternatives: 1) to turn the entire matter over to the Justice Department for prosecution—he stated that there were 26 or 27 counts on which this could be done; 2) to send me a letter by the end of the next week, officially blacklisting me; or, 3) to do nothing.

"He said that after careful consideration he had decided to issue a letter blacklisting me as an investigator for new drugs. Then he sat back and waited to see my reaction."

This, Jacob believed, was the cue for the victim to throw in the towel—to cry Uncle—to say blacklisting would be just fine and dandy with him.

Jacob said, "I advised Dr. Goddard that no self-respecting scientist or teacher could allow him to attempt to blacken his name without effective retaliation. I mentioned I would consult with the university administration and with my attorney. I said, 'If you carry out your threat, I will seek redress through the courts.'"

Something had gone wrong. Goddard had offered an amicable

solution to a messy problem. Justice was a simple thing when it involved only a couple of consenting adults.

"Dr. Goddard seemed surprised," Jacob's account continued. "I think he expected me to accept his proposal. He became angry and mentioned that perhaps he had made a mistake, maybe he *should* turn the entire matter over to the Department of Justice. I told him if this was what he wanted to do, he should go ahead.

"Dr. Goddard said he thought I wanted to become a martyr."

Jacob said that at this point he and Goddard went into a discussion of the merits of DMSO.

"Dr. Goddard does not know the literature on this drug," Jacob reported. "He had only superficial knowledge of what has been done. . . . I told this to Dr. Goddard; and I pointed out that, contrary to Dr. Hodges' statement that no drug company had submitted a formal request to release DMSO as a prescription item, three companies had done so—Merck, Syntex and Squibb.

"Since we did not seem to be making any progress," Jacob said, "the meeting came to an end. We shook hands."

Goddard told Jacob that he would receive an official statement blacklisting him by the twenty-sixth of May. It never came to pass.

Dr. Richard Brobyn, a smart young physician and general surgeon of Maple Grove, Pennsylvania, had worked out a bold plan to test DMSO's safety. As a consultant to Merck, he devised two regimens to be tested on volunteers—a short-term protocol covering two weeks, and a long one which would go on for three months.

Under this plan, the subjects would be given ten times the permissible dose of DMSO. Every single day, for two weeks. And if there were no serious effects from that, for three months.

When the FDA stopped virtually all experiments with DMSO, Merck lost its interest in DMSO and further human tests. But not Brobyn. He persisted. He presented his plan to Squibb and got them interested.

Squibb proposed that the FDA join them as partners in the venture. They would share the costs. The FDA agreed.

After two years of repeated promises to permit DMSO to be tested "properly," of contending the drug had shown severe toxic effects but refusing in each case to offer specific references, of saying doctors were still treating patients experimentally but declining to say where or who or on whom, of insisting that adequately equipped physicians could resume treating their patients but refusing to admit publicly that producers and distributors of DMSO were reluctant to accept the FDA's terms—after all this, the FDA finally gave Squibb and Brobyn permission for a controlled test of the drug for safety.

One October evening, in 1967, a group of sixty-seven healthy male prisoners at the California Medical Facility in Vacaville lined up in a large chilly hallway. They stripped, hung their clothes over chairs, and covered themselves from head to toe with a colorless gel—DMSO. Another thirty-three volunteers stripped but were untreated, because they were controls.

After two weeks of regular plasterings with DMSO, the procedures were stopped. The extensive examinations—including spinal taps, bone marrow punctures, eye studies, EKG for heart function, EEG for brain performance, and numerous tests of the blood, urine and other body fluids—were made again for the last time.

Examining physicians declared that the drug trials had been satisfactory; no prisoner-volunteer had shown evidence of a serious toxic effect of the drug. The ninety-day trials began.

The second group, of sixty experimental subjects and twenty controls, represented what the examining physicians described as "the largest and most competent toxicological study ever undertaken." The test subjects received ten times the ordinary therapeutic dose day in and day out; they were inspected and otherwise tested regularly—and so were the control subjects. Each man was paid $300 for his part in the study.

During the first three or four weeks, about twenty experimental subjects and a few of the controls dropped out. They had several reasons: 1) They didn't like the body odor DMSO induced or, in some cases, skin reactions; 2) they were not being rewarded enough; or 3) they went free or were moved to other prisons. On the other hand, several continued the test despite transient headaches and repeated skin reactions.

When the three months were over, Dr. Brobyn and his ophthalmologist partner, Dr. Frank Hull of Fairfield, California, filed an abstract on their findings. It said in part:

"This study plus monkey data at up to one hundred times the therapeutic dose for over a year have shown that the lens change is species specific and does not occur in primates. [Man, monkeys, apes and lemurs are primates.] Future areas of study based on the premise that DMSO is an extremely safe drug are listed."

Dr. Brobyn told me, "Of course, DMSO is a safe drug. I don't think there's any doubt about it. It did exactly what we intended . . . right to the letter."

Dr. Hull, the ophthalmologist, said there was no eye toxicity. Or, for that matter, no other serious side effects either. Don Wood, who had reported DMSO's effects on rabbit eyes, agreed that the human subjects showed no impairment.

The side effects were the same as those reported during the past five years by hundreds of doctors. Oyster odor of the skin and a garlic halitosis were common. The skin irritation was not rare, but most of those who experienced it went right on taking their DMSO. Headaches occasionally came and went. At ten times the ordinary dose, DMSO was amazingly gentle.

There were a few unexpected dividends. One man reported that his chronic back pain, which had required the removal of two spinal discs, had decreased. Another, whose ankle had been painfully stiff since a 1961 automobile accident, felt relief. Some said their postnasal drip and sinus conditions were better or their bursitis disappeared. The tests were for safety, however, not efficacy.

The Vacaville tests vindicated DMSO as no other drug in all

history had been vindicated of all suspicion of immediate toxic effects.

Hull and Brobyn examined the subjects for many months after the end of the study—Brobyn flew from Pennsylvania to California fourteen times that year. FDA investigators dropped in three times during the course of the study; and Stanley Jacob and one or two other investigators stopped by occasionally to chat with Hull, Brobyn and some of the prisoners.

The study cost $90,000, and this was split between the FDA and Squibb. It probably could be described as a classic in toxicology.

While the experiments gave DMSO a clean bill of health, so far as safety was concerned, nothing really came of them.

At 12:50 P.M., February 5, 1968, E. Rottenberg of the Ozothine Laboratories, Hauts-de-Seine, France, applied for a patent for DMSO "for treatment of all irritating conditions of the alimentary canal."

"By irritating conditions of the alimentary canal," the application stated, "one understands as included gastritis, duodenitis and colitis, acute and chronic, of all origins and all types, accompanied or not by ulcers."

Rottenberg's prescription was 4 per cent DMSO three times a day—or the equivalent of three times 60 mg of 100 per cent DMSO—taken orally as syrup, drops, tablets or another form.

He cited as support for his application these examples:

ACUTE GASTRITIS—Twenty-eight patients unable to work went back to their labors following five to eight days of treatment, rid of such symptoms as nausea, vomiting, pain, gastric heaviness; their stomach secretions became normal and so did their general condition. One year later, twenty-one were still free of symptoms, working and off their diets. During this time about ten had undergone treatment again for about fifteen days.

CHRONIC GASTRITIS—Thirteen patients on assorted treatments all relapsed on stopping treatment. On DMSO by mouth for one to two months, symptoms cleared up and all of them went back to work. At the end of a year, all of them remained improved, although some had resumed treatment two or three times.

PEPTIC ULCER—Five patients were completely cured of recent peptic ulcers with oral DMSO, without recurrence during the following year.

ENTERO-COLITIS—Six patients with abdominal pain for several months and with diarrhea, emaciated and asthenic, began to improve after eight days on oral DMSO, and all were back at work in two months, pain-free and in good shape.

MUCOMEMBRANOUS COLITIS—Three patients were "cured" after three weeks of oral DMSO.

When the DMSO is combined with star anise, the appetite improves, the application stated.

At this time, nothing had been heard from the U. S. Patent Office about the patents applied for six years earlier in Jacob's and Herschler's names for the state of Oregon and Crown Zellerbach.

One of the authorities on the history of DMSO was Dr. William Monte Hearon.

Hearon won his Ph.D. at MIT. He knew science—especially chemistry—and technology and business. He combined these aptitudes a few years after the end of World War II when he got a job with Crown Zellerbach on the chemistry of waste materials in paper and pulp products, a field in which Crown was a world leader. Hearon's job was twofold: 1) to transmute the base wastes into gold; and 2) make the stockholders rich.

This was before science and the press had discovered ecology and environment, and Crown showed little if any interest in eliminating its effluents and affronts to the several senses of innocent bystanders—the great, ugly gashes across the wooded hills and mountains where miles of trees were cut to satisfy America's appetites for news, pornography and literature, the dunes of sawdust that stood as a dusty monument to dead forests, the stench from log-choked waterways, the wind-swept fumes which turned vast areas of the blue sky into a ghastly yellow-gray, the massive timber and paper trucks that, like herds of panic-stricken elephants, stampeded along the highways, their engines shattering the calm of the day and the stillness of the night. (Recently, the engines have been muffled.)

His job was important to Hearon, and he did it well. He became Assistant Director of Research, and then General Manager of the Chemical Products Division, which he organized, put on a paying basis and ran for five years. He was sought out by Crown's biggest officers, brought into their important conferences, and on merit alone, given privileges within the Crown community that normally were reserved for those at the top of the payroll.

Hearon had civic and social interests, as well. He and his wife were quiet but indefatigable crusaders for disadvantaged people; they were active in church affairs; they were thoughtful toward each other and perhaps to everyone they knew, and they defended some who have many challengers but few champions.

When the FDA was at its toughest—and when Crown, coincidentally, was at its most timid—Hearon resigned. He had served Crown for twenty years. Since he had been Herschler's boss and bore some responsibility for the DMSO development, people asked, "Did he fall? Or had he been pushed?"

Hearon told me, "In 1958, we decided to build a big plant in Bogalusa, Louisiana, and we did. Then along about 1962, I formed the Chemical Products Division. I wanted Bob Herschler to think up new uses for the chemicals we could produce. And that's the job I gave him.

"Bob would dream up a hundred ideas and check them out at the lab to see if any were good. If they weren't, we'd forget them. If they were, we'd follow up.

"One of Bob's ideas was to use DMSO as a carrier of other materials—a control agent—in plants. He had a little greenhouse, and he tried it out. It worked. He reasoned: if DMSO will transport things in a plant or tree, shouldn't it work in animals or human beings?

"That's the kind of research he couldn't do for himself. It was fortunate that Stanley Jacob wanted DMSO as an antifreeze to preserve organs. Bob and Stan got together. And then things took off."

Hearon said that while Crown made improvements, the basic production patents used belonged to the Swedes who had developed them.

"There was general interest in DMSO at Crown," he said. "The real interest came later when we could file an IND (Investigational New Drug) application, and we could do some clinical work.

"I was much more optimistic than my colleagues. DMSO sounded unreal to them. Crown's feeling was: Okay, even if DMSO works as a drug and we produce ten thousand pounds of it a year, so what? In any good-sized mill, paper is produced in terms of thousands of tons a day.

"My own sentiments were entirely different. I thought of sick people and the help DMSO might give them.

"There are thirty-nine million pounds of aspirin produced and sold in the United States each year. If you were to substitute DMSO for aspirin, you'd be selling to a sizable market. And this is only for the kind of pain you use aspirin for."

He said that while there was no conclusive evidence that DMSO will cure any life-threatening disease, "We haven't begun to learn all of DMSO's uses."

Why did Crown knuckle under to the FDA?

"Crown is a paper company," he said. "It has never wanted to go into the drug business. We were deluged with inquiries from the public, problems of licensing, FDA approval, marketing. Crown didn't want this. And then the federal agents moved in and scared us. Crown panicked.

"I know Crown very well. The people who run it are extremely conscientious. They try to obey all the laws. They don't do any-

174

thing underhanded or on the fuzzy edge. They want to keep out of trouble, of course."

Hearon said he resigned from Crown "because I wanted to get into a business of my own. I got fed up with corporate life."

Had the FDA's tough attitude discouraged him from peddling DMSO as an industrial solvent?

"Crown is co-operating with the FDA," he said. "It has instituted certain controls."

Now that Crown was so well within the law, did FDA agents still visit their facilities?

"They come around two or three times a year," Hearon said. "Always unannounced. They look at the records and ask questions. Crown's lawyers are present. Crown makes every effort to give them what they want. Crown has been very diligent and very sensitive in being square with the law and all the regulations. We knocked ourselves out doing the right thing."

No one cognizant of the perils in the everyday practice of medicine, in the prescriptions filled in the corner drugstore, in the cosmetics, in the food we buy at the supermarket, in the toys, and gadgets, and gimmicks, and pots and pans, can deny that Goddard and the FDA had a difficult job—yes, some said an impossible job. And no one is more ready to admit this than FDA personnel themselves.

In some respects, Goddard was a godsend to the agency. He gave its personnel a purpose, a mission, a *raison d'être*.

Lean, wiry, with close-cropped prematurely gray hair, jutting jaw and eyes that searched warily from under bushy brows, this angry Irishman from Ohio looked and played the part of manning the last outpost of public health in a dirty and dangerous world. He was the defender of the law, protector of the people in a jungle overridden by wicked and cunning malefactors—microbe merchants, dream peddlers, nightmare dispensers, mind expanders, poison manufacturers, vitamin-crazy food faddists, drug hucksters, incompetent civil servants, conniving Congressmen, stupid scientists, unfit doctors, whining patients, meddlesome educators, lying writers and unconscionable editors.

Goddard built up a police force of three hundred agents, many schooled earlier, as T-men or G-men, to deal with desperate felons. He had a large staff of people who on Madison Avenue would be called press agents or publicity men but who were known in government under the euphemism "Information and Education Bureau."

Officers who were growing old in the service of the FDA, like his canny counsel Billy Goodrich, and a large supporting cast, could and did help him put together a tour de force rare in bureaucracy.

Goddard was unpredictable; and whether he was aware of it or not, this quality keeps a public figure in the news. He did not oppose the Administration's efforts to make LSD possession a federal offense, but neither did he show enthusiasm for it. He was quoted as telling a Senate Subcommittee on Juvenile Delinquency that while he regarded the hallucinogen as dangerous, "it would be unwise to provide penalties which might mark a large number of young people as criminals" merely because they had LSD for personal use. Some citizens complained that he uttered no such tolerance toward DMSO.

Goddard was willing to admit at least a few of his major errors. He had wanted skilled and dedicated workers around him, so he told all FDA employees at the start of his administration that they had a choice of doing a good job for him or getting out. A lot of able people, having no trouble finding employment in other bureaus, got out; he was left with the self-seeking inner circle who had always run the agency, with some stumblebum scientists and with hangers-on, along with ordinary workers.

He shuffled and reshuffled his top command, seeking effective innovations; and, as investigative committees later commented, the same old people, bearing new titles, popped up in the same positions of power, where they operated in the same old way.

On two occasions, he was quoted in ways that led his critics to charge that he was soft on dope. One quote was, "I believe we should not make a felony case against a young person for possession of marijuana. Marijuana is comparable to alcohol in its dangers when it comes to driving motor vehicles or operating heavy equipment." The other remark attributed to him was, "Whether or not it [marijuana] is more dangerous than alcohol is debatable. I don't happen to think that it is." Goddard charged that these observations had been taken out of context. While a good many authorities later echoed these sentiments, they were considered revolutionary when Goddard is said to have uttered them. He explained that he would object if any of his three college-age children used marijuana, because, he said, the long-term genetic effects had not been worked out, and there was a law against smoking it.

On various occasions, Goddard said something to injure the sensibilities of almost everybody. Some romantics and professionals were offended when he declared "the corner drugstore should be closed down"; he explained later that he was "talking about a long-term development—twenty years." Eyebrows went up when Goddard, a heavy cigarette smoker, on one occasion discussed the soaring lung cancer rate without mentioning cigarettes. "Is it all due to air [pollution]?" he asked. "We don't know for sure—but our suspicions are aroused."

His critics dusted off and applied to Goddard the diagnosis "foot-in-mouth disease."

Commissioner Goddard was good at giving punishment. He also had to take it.

Here is a small sample of opinions of Goddard's agency:

Written Consent. The American Medical Association charged that his edict requiring doctors to obtain the patient's written consent for treatment with investigational drugs "exceeds the authority delegated to the Commissioner, contains ambiguities which would result in confusion concerning the legal responsibilities of physicians, and is unwarranted interference with the practice of medicine."

Scientific Freedom. Dr. Michael B. Shimkin, a brilliant scientist, once the able medical director of the National Cancer Institute and at this time vice-president in charge of Temple University's flowering research program, said that the policies of the FDA (and the U. S. Public Health Service as well) were "uncomfortably reminiscent of the unhappy McCarthy era." "There is a need for a code of rights for the clinical investigator, including the right of appeal and defense, with confrontations against accusations that are made openly or by innuendo, on the basis of which penalties can be exacted for unfounded charges," he said.

Nutrition. Goddard and the FDA proposed this label on vitamin bottles: "Vitamins and minerals are supplied in abundant quantities in the foods we eat. The Food and Nutrition Board of the National Research Council recommends that dietary needs be satisfied by foods. Except for persons with special medical needs, there is no scientific basis for recommending routine use of supplements." The august National Research Council promptly denounced this startling pronouncement as "objectionable and misleading."

Delay. Goddard publicly vowed he would clean up the FDA's notorious backlog of applications for approval of new drugs. He did, technically—by turning much of the job over to 150 doctors and pharmacists from other agencies, approving slightly altered versions of old familiar drugs, and "pingponging" 130 proposals back to manufacturers for fuller information, the equivalent of sweeping them under the rug.

Errors of Omission. Dr. Maurice B. Vischer, Professor of Physiology at the University of Minnesota, explained FDA negativism this way: "No civil servant is as vulnerable to criticism for delays which might in the end sacrifice thousands of lives as he would be for positive action that cost one life."

And Commission. FDA approval of a new anti-flu drug, amantadine hydrochloride, was described as "dangerous" and "unthinkable" by Dr. Albert Sabin, developer of the oral polio vaccine, and Nobelist Dr. John Enders.

Truth. When Goddard's FDA alleged that one third of the members of the Pharmaceutical Manufacturers Association had violated the agency's advertising regulations, C. Joseph Stetler,

PMA President, asked, "Isn't it fair to require that an agency which demands the truth deliver the truth?"

Censorship and Dictatorship. Dr. Walter Modell, Professor of Pharmacology at Cornell University Medical College, was the author of a widely reprinted editorial, "FDA Censorship," in the journal *Clinical Pharmacology and Therapeutics*, which he edits:

> The FDA has now taken the stand that in this country it is the sole arbiter of drug dosage and that its pronouncements on this subject in drug package stuffers are inviolate. It has already acted to prevent authors from publishing articles citing dosages (not coinciding with those approved by FDA). No writing on therapy will be more expert than that of the group of nonexperts in the FDA. . . . The implications of this unprecedented FDA program are shattering.
>
> When the nonexpert ingroup of the FDA threatens to become the dictator of American medicine, we believe it will lead medicine from its present eminence to its ultimate decline. The best we can expect now is therapeutic nihilism.
>
> Where may a physician publicly disagree with the FDA on matters of dosage? Once the precedent of censorship is established, who is to say where it will end?
>
> The Public is protected by existing legislation against irresponsible errors by publishers, editors, and authors. Who will protect the public against the FDA?
>
> To hold scientists and physicians in jeopardy if they dare disagree publicly with the FDA is against all the canons of science and scholarship. In our opinion, it is in the worst interests of our nation's health; it is a barrier to education; and it is for no one's welfare.

Professional and public opinion were beginning to close in on Goddard and the FDA. One committee within the FDA and another outside it were gathering information on the agency. A growing number of doctors were defying Goddard and the laws he professed to enforce. As professional rebellion grew, bureaucratic strictures relaxed. The FDA once again seemed to be on a recidivous course back to its familiar state of futility and apathy.

Twenty-eight months after taking the job, Goddard resigned as FDA commissioner. He cited "personal reasons" to HEW Secretary Wilbur J. Cohen as the cause of his departure; and Cohen, in accepting the resignation, paid him the compliments usually awarded a public servant who quits under non-scandalous circumstances. Some speculated that the Johnson administration couldn't take any more of Goddard's "activist" behavior in an election year; some said he was physically and emotionally tired of the binds he found himself in, many of them of his own creation. Others said that he was being passed over for promotion. In any event, he was picking up his fat federal pension and retiring to the vice-presidency of EDP Technology, Inc., based in his wife's old hometown, Atlanta, Georgia.

In his swan song—an address before the AMA's American College of Legal Medicine in San Francisco, June 16, 1968—he defended his finding several clinical investigators ineligible and stated that "this kind of surveillance continues"; he said that the finding of "less than a dozen investigators who have raised suspicions" ought not to loosen confidence in the ability of clinicians generally as investigators "given proper orientation and guidance."

"The rascals will be exposed," he said, "even though their signboards may remain untouched over their office doors for periods longer than we can tolerate." He castigated the lawyers in his audiences for inadequately defending the nation's poor; and he charged the nation's doctors with failing all classes. He denied categorically charges that his administration was leading to "therapeutic nihilism" ("Professional nihilism comes through as the message," he said), or that the FDA had imposed censorship on the medical profession. And as for the package insert, he insisted that it should not be viewed as a mandate from the FDA's "non-expert in-group or as the dogma of drug therapy," but rather as the result of a thirty-year-old law requiring directions for drug use and "an aid to physicians who want to know how to use the drug it has accompanied, and it is the only FDA-approved public record of what we know about the safety and efficacy of the drug."

Goddard also defended his crusade for a Drug Compendium, the mock-up of which was big city telephone book size. A critic, Dr. Louis Lasagna, had said one version of it sounded like "a modern five-foot shelf of package inserts," and he expressed apprehension that such a volume would curtail the doctor's practice of good medicine.

Goddard's valedictory could be interpreted as a bitter denunciation of men like Modell and Lasagna who had challenged his bid for power over the practice of medicine and who had helped put him down in defeat.

Part Three

Goddard's successor as commissioner was Herbert L. Ley, Jr., M.D.

Ley was graduated, cum laude, from Harvard Medical School in 1946 and became Chairman of the Department of Microbiology in the Harvard School of Public Health. He had done stints on the faculty of George Washington University School of Medicine and in the sciences branch of the Army, before taking a job with the FDA at age forty-four. He was a large man, industrious, approachable, and, in a preoccupied, professorial way, amiable.

I talked with Ley on the afternoon of St. Valentine's Day 1969, in his office—Goddard's old headquarters. J. Kenneth Kirk, the Associate Commissioner of Compliance, sat in.

From the outset, Ley made it clear that his conduct of the office would differ from Goddard's. He said, "Dr. Goddard is one unique type person; he had done many things that it would be difficult for me to do as an individual. I'm another personality type. I am less flamboyant than Dr. Goddard. I think that there may be some things I can do perhaps better in my way than he could do. I am strongly committed personally to a full, fair but firm enforcement of the statutes which guide us as a nation."

My principal mission was to nail down, if possible, any evidence of severe DMSO toxicity. Reasonable proof that DMSO had killed or seriously harmed people would tend to justify the agency's extreme delay in releasing the drug.

I asked Ley if he shared Goddard's assumption that DMSO was highly toxic.

The commissioner was given to answering some questions with small speeches which were not entirely responsive. In due course, he came to this part: "There are possibilities of various types of hypersensitivity reactions, some of which have been documented in the literature, which may be quite severe, leading to death in a few people—"

I interrupted here: "Do you recall where this was reported, Doctor?"

He answered: "The reports are in our files here, and I do not have this information at our fingertips. But in a review of the whole file a year ago, the hypersensitivity type of reaction is a rare one with DMSO. But it obviously does occur."

This was the sort of thing that Jacob, Rosenbaum, Brobyn, Wood, Scherbel, Brown and all who were most familiar with DMSO feared and, in a way, expected, an allergic reaction, with the collapse of blood vessels, chaotic spasms of the pulmonary and digestive systems, convulsions, and, very often, sudden death. It was what they feared, but what had never come to pass. The massive and still mounting medical literature on DMSO showed no reaction stronger than a mild and fleeting histamine release syndrome. The drug seemed to have a clean slate after millions of DMSO treatments.

"You say there have been several deaths due to hypersensitivity reactions to DMSO?" I asked. I had to be sure.

"This is apparently the case," Ley said. He said the evidence was incorporated in a "white paper" prepared a year earlier, and he promised me a copy soon. I hoped it would be more specific and informative than the "white papers" I had seen. He, and Kirk as well, had no idea how many patients were under experimental treatment with DMSO.

I mentioned the apprehension incited by FDA agents' "visits."
"We have had no reason to pursue this type of approach within
the past year," Ley said. "There's been no stimulus for it."

Ley and Kirk both denied vigorously that the FDA had blacklisted scientists. Ley described in several hundred words precisely
what had been done to scientists, and the actions he described
met, in every detail, what I would consider the dictionary definition of blacklisting.

I asked whether Ley had changed the procedure, and he answered, "We changed it by adding the second level of review."

When I brought up the damage done by this type of character
assassination, it occurred to Ley that we were running out of the
time allotted to me. Both men suggested that if I had further
questions and would write them out and mail them in, they'd be
glad to answer them.

I left the Ley interview, as I had the Goddard interview, per-
plexed that these high officials seemed so lacking in solid information about the most spectacular and the most controversial
drug of our time and, as Congressman Wyatt had expressed it, a
"persecuted drug."

Not only did the FDA lack data to support its charge that
DMSO was forbiddingly toxic but it was proving amazingly un-
informed on the results of laboratory and clinical studies. At this
time, the proceedings of the New York Academy and the Vienna
meetings had been published and many papers were being repub-
lished in various journals. There also was a strong surge of scientific reports, mainly from abroad, flatly suggesting that DMSO
was indeed a "wonder drug," and one without great toxicity.

Following are a few of the many reports available to alert
agencies, as I have boiled them down:

ATHLETIC INJURIES

A total of 47 athletes were treated for sports-associated conditions
—30 of them with acute sprains, strains, dislocations, serious cuts

and the like, 7 of them with the syndromes which follow long immobilization for broken bones, and 10 for tennis elbow and other chronic conditions considered the result of a long series of "microtraumas." A wide range of sports were included—gymnastics, track and field events, Greco-Roman and conventional wrestling, football, tennis, basketball, judo, diving, swimming, weight-lifting, skiing, cycling, water polo and fencing.

The patients were treated three times a day for two days and twice a day thereafter by dabbing or pouring 90 per cent DMSO on the affected areas.

In cases of acute trauma, pain was relieved rapidly, sometimes spectacularly, swelling subsided, and function was recovered—"so spectacularly as to compel us to urge our patients to observe greatest caution in order to avoid further damage to a joint" which may not have healed completely.

Chronic conditions, some of which had become acute again, also responded rapidly with relief of pain, reduced swelling and increased function. DMSO also promoted rapid recovery and return to action following immobilization for fractures.

"The complete absence of undesirable collateral reactions, its ease of application, and the few precautions that should be observed make it (DMSO) a medication for wide use in medical therapy, and also an urgently needed medication in sports-related traumatology." [A. Venerando et al., Institute of Sports Medicine, Italy, *Gazz. Int. Med. Chir.* 70:1605 (1965)]

MUSCULOSKELETAL CONDITIONS

Fifteen patients with arthritis (rheumatoid), muscle pain or neuralgia which had persisted anywhere from one month to 20 years were treated with 90 per cent DMSO for from 12 to 20 days. Relief of pain was achieved in a mean of 10.2 minutes and lasted from 8 to 24 hours. DMSO also relieved edema and muscular spasm and improved function. Transient skin redness and halitosis were common. [E. U. Villarino, Mexicali, Baja California, *Revista Medicina* (Mexico), Vol. 45 (1965)]

ARTHRITIS AND RHEUMATISM

DMSO was applied to the affected areas of 37 patients—15 with rheumatoid arthritis, 9 with osteoarthritis, 7 with gout, and 6 with non-articular rheumatism. In more than 50 per cent of the patients, the results were excellent or good—there was unquestionable anti-inflammatory and pain-relieving effects. The side effects were slight and brief in all but two in whom the local reaction forced suspension of treatment; in both, however, an excellent response already had occurred. All patients had been resistant to other therapy. [M. M. Kalb, Mexico, D.F., *Medicina*, October 25, 1965]

ANTI-BACTERIAL EFFECT

DMSO in concentrations between 2.5 and 20 per cent was tested against a wide spectrum of bacteria. In these low strengths, DMSO did not kill the bacteria, but it did inhibit the growth of strains of Staphylococcus, Pseudomonas and E. coli. DMSO sensitized bacteria to antibiotics and other drugs to which they always had been or recently had become resistant.

DMSO in these concentrations inhibited the growth of these organisms: Gonococcus, 5 per cent; Pneumococcus, Corynebacterium diphtheriae, Streptococcus, 15 per cent; Pseudomonas, 10 per cent; and Staphylococcus, 10–20 per cent. The tests were carried out in bacterial cultures.

Eyeballs could be preserved for later transplantation in DMSO, aqueous humor and glycerin. The material was maintained in a refrigerator. [Sadayoshi Kamiya et al., Ophthalmology Dept., Nara College School of Medicine, *Jap. Jnl. of Clinical Ophthalmology* 20(2) (1966)]

LACK OF ANTI-BACTERIAL EFFECT

DMSO, in concentrations up to 10 per cent, did not alter the susceptibility of many bacteria to assorted antibiotics. Among the organisms tested were *Salmonella paratyphi, Proteus vulgaris, Pseudomonas aeruginosa, Streptococcus faecalis*, beta hemolytic Streptococcus group A, *Diplococcus pneumoniae, E. coli* and *Aerobacter cloacae*. Among the agents tested in these cultures were high and low concentrations of penicillin, erythromycin, chloromycetin, novobiocin, tetracycline, and dihydrostreptomycin.

While DMSO in low concentration neither reduced nor enhanced the action of drugs, in concentrations of 30 per cent and more it seemed to dissolve susceptible microorganisms. [Glenn E. Pottz et al., Greenville (S.C.) General Hospital, *Annals N. Y. Academy of Sciences*, Vol. 141 (March 15, 1967): 261–72]

VACCINES

DMSO (22–45 per cent) alone protected mice against typhus infection about as well as did an oral typhus vaccine—about 40 per cent protection. Combined, the two offered 47 per cent protection.

The Salk vaccine alone and the Salk vaccine plus DMSO offered about the same protection to mice—only 18 per cent of the mice succumbed to polio infection following vaccination, as compared with 50 per cent of the unvaccinated controls. There was one interesting difference, however: polio antibodies were found in mice given only the Salk vaccine but not in those given the combination.

DMSO had no effect on typhus vaccine given rabbits. [Hansjurgen Raettig, Robert Koch Institute, Berlin, Second International Symposium on DMSO, Vienna, November 1966]

EAR

A simple but painful operation is puncturing the eardrum to release pus and pressure from the inner or middle ear and introduce medicines to combat infection or other disease conditions. Some doctors elect to let their patients suffer the lesser pains of otitis rather than subject them to the pain of operation.

"While DMSO had had a bad name" recently, it had solved the problem in 107 patients with serous otitis and 50 with purulent otitis media. A single drop of DMSO was swabbed on the eardrums for one minute; it and an anesthetic, tetracaine hydrochlorida, made it possible to puncture the eardrum. None of the patients had severe pain; four out of five had no pain at all, and the rest slight pain. [Irving L. Ochs, of Annapolis, Md., at American Academy of Ophthalmology and Otolaryngology annual meeting, 1966]

INFLAMMATION

Rats were injected with turpentine. This caused the accumulation of fluid and a rise in their body temperature.

Intramuscular DMSO, in either 10 per cent or 100 per cent concentration, reduced the edema by 30 per cent. The dilute DMSO reduced the body temperature rise (0.4°C) by 0.16°, while concentrated DMSO brought it down 0.32°.

DMSO also prevented the ill effects of sunburn in exposed humans. [L'vov Scientific Conference, July 1–5, 1966, pp. 337–39, *Iu. N. Turkevich*, L'vov State Medical Institute]

COLD SORE

It took untreated cold sores of the lip (herpes labialis) 8.73 days to heal. The healing time was reduced to 5.67 days when DMSO was injected into the lesion with a Dermojet gun, and to 3.5 days (as compared with 9.8 days for controls in this series) when idoxuridine (IDU) in a 5 per cent DMSO solution was used. [F. D. MacCallum and B. E. Juel-Jensen of Oxford, *BMJ*, October 1, 1966]

ATHLETIC INJURIES

DMSO was applied to injuries of about 100 UCLA athletes during 1965 until November, when it was banned. DMSO proved of "great value" not only in major sports (UCLA won four national championships that year) but in minor sports as well. [Dr. Roderick Turner, UCLA team physician, N. Y. Academy of Sciences Conference on DMSO, 1966]

CREEPING ERUPTION

DMSO alone was applied to creeping eruptions on the skin of patients, and it proved of no benefit.

When DMSO in combination with 2 per cent thiabendazole was applied to creeping eruptions in 25 patients, all eruptions cleared up completely within three weeks. Thiabendazole, an anti-warm preparation, was dissolved in 90 per cent DMSO in these double blind experiments. [Drs. Robert Katz and Robert W. Hood, Univ. of Miami, Fla., at AMA meeting in Chicago, June 1966]

DERMATOLOGICAL CONDITIONS

A combination of the cortisone-type hormone, fluocinolone acetonide, 0.025 per cent, and 90 per cent DMSO was tested over a period of one year in 174 patients with 32 different dermatological conditions.

No serious side effects were noted in any patient. "Outstanding results" were obtained in a majority of cases of acne vulgaris, granuloma annulare, herpes zoster, postzoster neuritis, lichen planus, lichen simplex chronicus, lupus erythematosus (discoid), and in a minority of cases or single cases of alopecia areata, chronic benign familial pemphigus, dermatitis herpetiformis, lichen sclerosis, molluscum contagiosum, morphea, poikiloderma atrophicans vasculare, and psoriasis. [Samuel Ayres, Jr., M.D., and Richard Mihan, M.D., UCLA and USC, respectively, *Cutis*, Vol. 3, No. 2 (February 1967)]

SCLEROMA

DMSO, as an aerosol, immediately penetrated into the tissues of scleroma patients and carried with them such antibiotics as streptomycin, terramycin, aureomycin and others with good results. As treatment proceeds, it may become necessary to use corticosteroids, oxygen, glucose transfusions, vitamins, codliver oil, iron and anti-histamines. [R. A. Bariliak and N. A. Sakhelashvili, *Voprosy Sanologii* (L'vov) (1967): 230–34]

URINARY CALCULI

One group of rats drank tap water. Another group drank water with 6 per cent DMSO—and when they lost weight because of the diuretic effect, the concentration was lowered to 3 per cent DMSO, on which they maintained normal weight. Both groups were fed a pelleted ration on which lambs had developed a high incidence of urinary calculi.

After two months, 40 of the 45 water-drinking rats had developed calculi of the kidney, bladder or ureter, while only 11 of the 46 DMSO group showed the calculi. Besides stones, the calculi also took the form of rubbery plugs, found mainly in the bladder. [Fu-ho

Chen Chow, et al., Colorado State Univ., *Journal of Urology*, February 1967]

DERMATOLOGY

DMSO yielded generally good results in 16 of 23 cases of keloid and hypertrophic scars, 1 in 3 of induratio penis plastica, 6 of 9 of Dupuytren's contracture of the hand, 3 of 4 in scleroderma, 17 of 21 of eczema tyloticum, 6 of 9 infiltrative processes of the lower limbs, 4 of 7 sclerodermic changes in post-thrombotic syndrome, 3 of 5 granuloma anulare, 3 of 4 lichen ruber verrucosus, 2 of 4 verrucae vulgaris, 4 of 4 combustio, 10 of 11 herpes zoster and post-zoster neuralgia, 0 of 2 fibroma—75 of a total of 106 patients.

Almost full recovery was noted in one scleroderma patient after six weeks of treatment, and considerable healing and improved mobility was observed in another patient who had had the disease 15 years. Local and general side effects were not serious enough to halt treatment. [H. Weitgasser, Gebietskrankenkasse, Graz; *Zschr. Haut Geschl.-Krkh.*, Vol. 42, 18 (1967): 749–54]

FUNGUS INFECTION

DMSO was mixed with antifungal preparations and used to treat seven patients with various kinds of fungus infections, including those of the finger and toe nails. Improvement sometimes started on the second day of treatment.

During application, there was noticed a light itch, a stitch feeling and a burning sensation, all of which disappeared within 20 to 30 minutes. Immediately after application, an edema appeared on three men and a tendency to form a blister on a woman.

While a final opinion can not be formed, it is advisable to continue the study of this remedy for fungoid diseases of the skin and nails. [J. M. Domantovskaya et al., Soviet Union; *Vest. Derm.* 2 (1967): 13–18]

RADIATION DAMAGE

Very high doses of cobalt radiation were delivered to 22 patients —15 with cancer of the ovary, 3 with breast cancers, and 4 with other cancers. Side effects included indurated scarring and ulcers.

All 22 patients were swabbed with DMSO, or had DMSO sprayed over the affected parts, two or three times a day. Two begged off further DMSO treatment because of sensations of tingling, burning and pain; the remaining 20 tolerated the DMSO well and were not disturbed particularly by the odor.

Six registered neither subjective nor objective improvement.

Fourteen showed objective improvement, including softening of the scars, increased movement of joints, and the clearing up of skin ulcers in all three patients who had them, including two who had had them for more than two years. [Prof. H. L. Köllinh, F. H. Glaser and M. Klaua, Martin Luther Univ., Halle-Wittenberg, *Rad. biol. ther.* 11/4]

WOUND HEALING

Rabbits were anesthetized and surgical wounds were inflicted along the backs. Some wounds were swabbed immediately and periodically thereafter with 70 per cent DMSO. All wounds then were sutured and the animals put in isolation. Sutures were removed on the fourth day, and the animals were killed and autopsied between then and the fourteenth day.

Scar tissue was removed and measured for its ability to withstand tension without rupturing.

No differences were observed in tissues of animals killed before the seventh day. Those killed from then on however registered striking differences: The scar tissue of the DMSO-treated rabbits was "very significantly" (one chance of error in 100) the stronger, possibly due to an increased blood supply to the superficial tissues. [Harold M. Albert of New Orleans and Nguyen Huu of Saigon, *La Presse Medicale*, January 7, 1967]

BENIGN BREAST DISEASE

Two series of women with mastopathy—benign breast disease—were treated in the Breast Clinic of Gynecological Hospital of the University of Heidelberg. The first group of 134 were all given DMSO, which they applied to their breasts once each night for several weeks. The second group of 129 were treated with DMSO or a placebo in a double blind test—neither the patient nor the physician knew who got what; this experiment ran for four weeks.

The patients were examined, questioned, and given mammography tests before and after the four-week course. They were graded for (slight, distinct or complete) relief of breast pain, shrinkage of swollen breasts, and decrease of tenderness. They were re-checked in the same manner two months after the end of the experiment to determine whether good results still persisted.

Of 75 women in the uncontrolled series who could be followed and subjected to a detailed physical and x-ray check-up, 52 showed subjective improvement (11 slight, 24 distinct, 17 complete). Of the 55 women reporting and showing objective improvement, x-rays showed healing and reduced swelling in the breasts in a great majority, with two-thirds of them reporting persisting improvement at the end of the study. And of 14 women who reported slight or no improvement after the last application of DMSO, 12 of them—12 of the 14—two months later came to report distinct relief or complete improvement, with ten of them showing objective signs of good results, as a delayed action effect of DMSO.

Of the 75 patients who reported for a check-up two months after treatment had stopped, only one had observed no side effects. Each time after treatment, 30 confirmed sensations of heat, odor, itching and/or tingling of the treated skin. Some of the skins had scaled, or blistered; almost all had had halitosis, which often vanished with teeth brushing. Cortisone-like hormones usually extinguished the most severe of these side effects. [H. Lau et al., Univ. of Heidelberg, *Deutsche Med. Wochensch.*, Vol. 93, No. 44 (1968)]

LIMB BLOOD VESSELS

Twelve patients with various disorders of the limb arteries, veins and lymphatic vessels were treated with 1) a spray of 15 per cent DMSO to facilitate penetration of other drugs through their ill-nourished skins, and 2) a 60 per cent DMSO ointment and tincture to treat inflammation resulting from their circulatory disease.

"The good results show the usefulness of DMSO in the treatment of arterial, venous and lymphatic disorders of the limbs." [A.

Kappert; Ang. Lab. Anna Seiler Hans Inselsp, Bern, *Schweiz. Med. Wschr.* 98 (46) (November 16, 1968)]

ANTI-VIRUS

Four RNA viruses (Influenza A and A_2, Newcastle disease and Semliki Forest) and two DNA viruses (vaccinia and E. coli phage T_2) lost their infectivity completely during 30 minutes of exposure to 80 per cent DMSO. DMSO concentrations of 60 per cent and lower were ineffective.

DMSO at 80 per cent was highly effective against a cancer (polyoma) virus and, at 60 to 80 per cent, against an influenza (PR-8) virus; but its anti-viral potency diminished rapidly as its concentration went down. Because DMSO destroys fungi, bacteria, and viruses, it would be a useful sterilizing agent where autoclaving is impossible. [James C. Chan and Hans H. Gadebusch, Squibb Institute for Medical Research, New Brunswick, N.J., *Applied Microbiology*, October 1968]

THYROID DEPRESSION

DMSO, at 5 and 15 per cent, depressed the activity (iodine uptake) of cultured mouse thyroids more effectively than did standard thyroid-depressing drugs (propylthiouracil and thiocyanate). The DMSO effect was reversed by simply washing the organ in water.

DMSO, at 63 per cent strength, exercised a small but significant thyroid suppressing effect when injected into mice. [Ronald F. Hagemann and Titus C. Evans, Radiation Research Laboratory, Univ. of Iowa College of Medicine, *Proc. Soc.* (1968): 1008–10]

BLADDER

When DMSO was painted on the pubic areas of 15 patients who had interstitial cystitis resistant to other therapy, only two were significantly improved.

When 50 per cent DMSO was instilled into the bladder and left there for 15 minutes, six of the eight patients so treated showed significant improvement; and all patients returned for this simple office procedure enthusiastically every two to four weeks. Most patients reported they "hadn't felt better in years."

When the FDA banned further treatment with DMSO, the patients returned reluctantly to their former treatment: endoscopic hydrodilation of the bladder under general anesthesia every two or three months along with chemofulguration, which afforded partial relief of symptoms. [Bruce H. Stewart, Lester Persky and William S. Kiser, Cleveland Clinic and Western Reserve Univ., *Journal of Urology*, December 1968]

DIURESIS

When 5 per cent DMSO was added to their drinking water, rats increased their urinary output to four or five times normal. Investigation of the hormone-producing parts of the brain indicated that the phenomenon was not due to enhanced synthesis and release of anti-diuretic hormone. [J. Suominen and S. Uusi-Pentila, Turku Univ., Finland, *Z Ges. Exp. Med.* 147 (1) (1968): 38–43]

THROMBUS FORMATION

Platelets are sticky little particles in the blood which 1) vulcanize ruptured vessels and minimize hemorrhage, and 2) which sometimes clump into plugs that stop up arteries and cause strokes and heart attacks.

Sixteen anti-inflammatory agents were tested for their suppressive effect on five different drugs which cause platelet clumping. DMSO, in only 1 per cent concentration, inhibited significantly every agent's ability to cause clumping, both in living animals and in laboratory dishes.

Even when applied on the hamster's cheek pouch, prior to administering a clumping agent (adenosine diphosphate, in this case), 1 per cent DMSO permitted clumps to form in only one of ten animals tested. [P. Görög and Iren B. Kovacs, United Pharmaceutical Works, Budapest, International Symposium on Inflammation Biochemistry, Como, Italy, October 1968]

HARD-TO-MANAGE DISEASES

Four series of 12 patients each were treated with DMSO—by spray and/or tincture, alone or with such drugs as rutin, linoleic acid or vitamin A—for painful and difficult-to-control diseases.

The response to therapy—subjective and objective—was graded Good, Moderate, or None. Subjective improvement included remission, or disappearance of pain, congestion and paresthesia. Objective meant remission, or healing of hardened tissue, and various skin manifestations of disease.

This is the box score of results—SUBJECTIVE:

	GOOD	MODERATE	NONE
Post-thrombotic syndrome (spray)	6	3	3
Scleroderma and related diseases (tincture)	4	5	3
Arterial occlusion conditions, Stages III & IV (spray or tincture)	5	3	4
Brachialgia of blood vessel origin & leg cramps (spray or tincture)	6	2	4

OBJECTIVE RESULTS

Post-thrombotic syndrome	3	5	4
Scleroderma and related diseases	3	3	6
Trophic disturbances in art. occlusion, etc.	4	4	4
Brachialgia, etc.		(No organic findings).	

[A. Kappert, Berne, *Schweiz. Med. Wschr.* 98 (46) (1968): 1829–37]

The Food and Drug Administration officials answered questions about DMSO with short stereotyped notes and one of two enclosures—a so-called "white paper" or a "fact sheet."

The "white paper," which ran variously between two and ten thousand words, may well become a museum piece in governmental communications. There is no signature to identify the author and no letterhead to indicate its FDA origins. It has never been presented before scientific or medical audiences. There are no data, no bibliography, no references, no author or agency with whom to check the statements of "fact."

The second type of enclosure, a "fact sheet," is presented under the FDA letterhead. It is a digest of the "white paper," with interchangeable phraseology, and equally anonymous, data-less, without references or identifiable or responsible sources. Scientists have disputed the innuendo, insinuations and many of the alleged facts in the "white paper" and the "fact sheet." Here is a version I have boiled down from the latest, most moderate, and most honest "white paper":

Interest in possible drug uses for DMSO in man accelerated rapidly from 1962 to 1965. In October, 1963, the first Notice of Claimed Investigational Exemption for a New Drug (IND) to provide for clinical testing of DMSO in humans was submitted. Also submitted were 3 New Drug Applications (NDA's) for commercial marketing of DMSO for drug use.

Preclinical Evaluation for Safety

Data from preclinical animal studies in the first investigation filed with the FDA failed to support the safety of DMSO for all the proposed clinical trials. The FDA recommended restricting the product to a very limited cutaneous study.

The data disclosed serious toxic signs in some animals, appearing at dose levels which suggested little or no margin of safety in humans. However, in other species the toxic manifestations appeared only at high dose levels. Some of the more serious adverse effects reported were hemolytic anemia, lesions of the gastrointestinal tract, liver, lung, and spleen; dilatation of nerve sheaths of brain and spinal cord; hematuria, abortions and teratogenic effects. In all animals corneal and lenticular changes of the eye were observed. These eye changes were more moderate and marginal in the monkey.

Concurrently, the results of DMSO testing in humans were evaluated. However, before a scientific opinion was reached, articles appeared in the popular press, representing DMSO as a "wonder" drug, for treatment of a variety of diseases. There were no adequate scientific data to justify these glowing accounts, but the publicity excited the interest of the medical profession and the laity. DMSO was readily available in many communities in commercial grades for industrial use and thus there was an easy and unrestricted source of supply.

An estimated more than 100,000 patients received DMSO during 1964 and 1965. Many of the clinical studies were poorly-designed and conducted, but claims of excellence were made on such uncontrolled studies.

The adverse effects of DMSO on the eyes of animals were manifested as change in the refractive index of the lens and by nuclear sclerosis. These adverse reactions were not disclosed to the FDA by responsible sponsors until November of 1965.

Reported cutaneous application of DMSO has disclosed a spectrum of allergic-like reactions, from generalized urticaria and respiratory distress to angioneurotic edema and anaphylaxis. Adverse experience involving the human eye are described by such phrases as "impaired vision of rather vague type," "decreasing vision," "bleary vision," "like wearing dark glasses," "vitreous opacity," "pain in one eye," "double vision," and "increased relucency."

Clinical testing was discontinued by voluntary agreement of all the sponsoring pharmaceutical firms and the FDA because of the question of safety.

On November 25, 1965, the FDA announced termination of clinical testing and investigational use of the drug, except in laboratory animals. Clinical testing with DMSO was not completely prohibited but, in the interest of patient safety, was strictly controlled.

During 1966 a comprehensive evaluation of all available data on DMSO indicated that further clinical investigation of the drug was justified for cutaneous application in serious conditions, such as scleroderma, persistent herpes zoster, and severe rheumatoid arthritis, for which no satisfactory therapy was available.

Between October 23 and November 6, 1967, a [14-day toxicity] study disclosed that, for treatment of relatively benign conditions, DMSO was reasonably safe; ophthalmological examinations were not necessary when cutaneous use of the drug was limited to 14 days. In the second phase, a 90-day study, adverse reactions were headache, pruritus, nausea, sedation, and dizziness. Examinations disclosed no demonstrable eye changes, but a small percent of subjects complained of hazy vision and burning sensation in the eye. In both phases of the study there was a tendency toward eosinophilia (histamine-type of response) and skin irritation during treatment.

DMSO appears to give temporary symptomatic relief in some patients with scleroderma. In our judgment the adverse reactions reports received do not appear to seriously jeopardize safety.

A government agency is the sponsor of a notice for use of DMSO as an endocellular cryophylactic agent in the process of freeze preservation of blood platelets for the infusion of blood elements into thrombocytopenic, leukopenic and aplastic anemia patients. These studies are being carried out in 5 medical centers under the government agency and at present approximately 100 patients are receiving such treatment. In addition, there are two independent clinical investigators conducting similar studies in other centers.

At present 21 sponsors of IND's are conducting clinical trials on a total of approximately 2404 patients in the treatment of acute and chronic conditions.

The "white paper" could have been the source for ever so many doctors. When the subject of DMSO came up, some doctors were likely to say with conviction, "DMSO? Very toxic, you know. Could blind a person. Hard on the liver too."

From this point, the dialogue usually went:

Q: Ever given DMSO to a patient?

A: No—can't say that I have.

Q: Ever use it yourself?

A: Never.

Q: Ever know anyone who was harmed by it?

A: No.

Q: Then how do you know it's risky?

A: It's right there in the literature. The FDA says so.

Many patients sent Stanley Jacob letters and accounts showing how their physicians had discouraged the use of DMSO, often on information from the FDA.

There was an exchange between Dr. Y and a labor union official. Dr. Y wrote: "The initial claims of success have not been substantiated by further investigation, and it is currently being used on a research basis only . . . most of the reports seem to indicate that it does have some value in acute muscular strains and sprains when applied to the skin . . . however it does have some side effects causing dehydration and loss of fat in the skin with dryness and flaking because of its powerful solvent action."

He then added: "As to the charge that the FDA is dragging its feet in approving it for general use, this does not appear justified to me. In some respects this situation is analagous to Krebiozen, the anti-cancer drug that had great claims made for its success but were not substantiated when placed in the hands of competent investigators. I have taken the liberty of checking with others who would be more knowledgeable in this field and they seem to concur in this evaluation."

Dr. Y made it clear—as so many critics of DMSO had before him—that "I have had no personal experience with it."

L. A. Healey, M.D., a director of the Arthritis Foundation of Western Washington, wrote in an article that he had tested DMSO, before the FDA ban, on patients with rheumatoid arthritis.

Healey wrote, in part:

> It was supposed to relieve pain and stiffness in joints and tendons, not only in acute inflammatory conditions like bursitis or sprains which are self-limiting and will in time clear up by themselves, but in chronic diseases such as rheumatoid arthritis as well. As is well known, there is no complete cure for rheumatoid arthritis and anything which seems to show promise naturally arouses great interest.
>
> There was some evidence of cataracts developing in animals given DMSO experimentally.
>
> Before it was withdrawn, I had the opportunity to try DMSO in patients with rheumatoid arthritis. I am sure it was not as good as was claimed. It gave temporary relief of joint pain but did not affect the swelling or joint inflammation. . . . I do not belittle this, as temporary relief is frequently welcome, but it was no cure for arthritis and did not appear to alter the disease process in the joints.

Healey complained that "headline writing, of course, is a separate art; closer related to the carnival barker at times than to the story itself."

The headline on Healey's handout was: "DMSO—ANOTHER 'MIRACLE' DRUG EVERYONE SHOULD AVOID NOW."

The spirit of the FDA reached beyond America's shores. It was felt keenly in Germany, where science, medicine and the pharmaceutical industry had come to reject the FDA. The trouble was, the FDA continued to sound its alarm through "white papers," "fact sheets" and the like, and no one dared openly dispute it. As a prescription drug, DMSO was sold with multiple restrictions as to dosage and administration routes; and the industry decided not to promote it. No drug can succeed without promotion.

Late in 1968, I wrote to Priv. Doz. Dr. med. Gerhard Laudahn, Director of Schering AG, in Berlin and asked how Germany was responding to the availability of DMSO.

"Much to my regret," he replied, "DMSO sales have not come up to my expectations.

"There is still the psychological handicap that soon after its introduction onto the market, DMSO had to be withdrawn and then was re-introduced more than a year later. Hence, there is still an attitude of reserve, and the preparation is still being very carefully observed."

Laudahn was satisfied with DMSO's performance as a drug.

"The expectations we placed in DMSO regarding its use in acute inflammatory conditions of the musculoskeletal system have been fully realized," he said. "As regards chronic conditions, such as rheumatic arthritis, scleroderma, etc., we have not come across any more information, since in Germany and Austria the use of DMSO is limited to 14 days."

He said that DMSO research in Germany had stagnated since "the severe set-back in the U.S.A.," meaning the FDA crackdown. He said that in Germany and the United States, "it may be that DMSO will not regain its original popularity unless completely new fields of application, such as cancer, for example, are opened."

I was not the only one who had difficulty getting solid information from the FDA. Paul de Haen of New York was having his troubles too.

A highly respected authority on the introduction of new drugs —or old drugs in new guises or new combinations—de Haen interprets developments for the pharmaceutical industry and others concerned with the drug trade throughout the world.

Near the end of February 1969, he told me that he had found it impossible to get essential statistics from the FDA.

He said the FDA did not differentiate between new drugs, single drugs, combination drugs that are newly marketed, and drug applications for variations of them, or for new uses for old drugs.

"You really never know what they have," he said.

The British, on the other hand, leveled. They gave honest figures.

In his annual review, *New Products Parade 1968*, de Haen reported that during the decade 1959–68, in the United States the total number of new drugs had declined from 315 (in 1959) to 87 (in 1968), the number of new single chemicals from 63 to 11, duplicate single products from 49 to 26, combination products from 203 to 50, and new dosage forms from 104 to 21.

In 1968, a majority of the new products introduced into the United States came from abroad; only three of the seven new original products, and one of the four other derivatives of old compounds were American. It was apparent too that researchers were publishing more and more about less and less—perhaps a progressive approach to the end point of writing everything about nothing. De Haen said he had harvested 5,780 reports on pharmaceutical specialties in 1968 as compared with 4,969 during the previous year.

Bad as 1968 had been, it was still much better than 1969. During the twelve months, the total number of new products dropped from 87 to 62; and the number of new single chemicals introduced in the United States declined from 11 to 9, with comparable cuts in other drug categories as well.

Despite its scientific decay, the drug industry prospered. Americans were buying more drugs (old ones, that is) than ever before, and the drug houses' profits were achieving new records each year. A pill hungry society would buy whatever was offered.

"Quadriplegia is the saddest thing that happens to people," Jacob said. "It occurs most often to the young and healthy—to soldiers fighting our wars, to youngsters driving, to athletes in personal contact games.

"As a quadriplegic, you lie in bed, a total vegetable, unable to move any of your extremities. Your mind functions, but you can't pass urine. You can't have a bowel movement without help. You are totally dependent upon someone else to perform the basic functions—to keep you alive."

I had asked who stood to gain most from DMSO.

"As I get to know the quadriplegics, ever so many of them eventually will say to me, 'You know, Dr. Jacob, I couldn't even commit suicide.' "

At this time, he was treating eight quadriplegics; and of them only one had presented a recently incurred injury. He felt, as do most doctors, that treatment is more fruitful in new than old conditions. The one fresh case was that of a sixteen-year-old girl, a fine athlete, who dove off a board and landed on her neck on the bottom of the pool.

"Her doctor was pessimistic but willing to try almost anything that offered a glimmer of hope. She was a complete quadriplegic —utterly helpless.

"She was on DMSO for an entire year. Gradually—one by one, it seemed—her organs began to function again. Eventually she walked. And now she is in college, doing very well."

It was 3:30 P.M. on Saturday, April 5, 1963. Grey Keinsley, eighteen, was driving from Greeley, where he was a freshman at the University of Northern Colorado, to Denver, where he was going to apply for a summer job with the State Highway Department. The Rocky Mountain sunshine and bracing air flooded through the open suntop of his VW, and it might have been that open top that saved his life. To this day he doesn't know what happened.

They lifted the athletic body off the barbwire fence where it had been hanging, limp and battered, and they took him, still breathing but unconscious, to the Community Hospital at Longmount. The doctor said, "Have this boy's family get here without delay."

The way it looked to the doctors: the numerous bruises and cuts would heal in time—if there was time. One could survive the concussion. But the broken neck was another thing; x-rays showed a fracture four over five, a spinal cord block between the cervical vertebrae four and five, a vital link in communications between the brain and the body below the neck.

When Grey heard his parents' voices, he came out of the coma momentarily, but he was delirious for weeks.

Mrs. Dorothy M. Keinsley of Littleton, Colorado, had told me of Grey's struggle. His father being in the U. S. Army, Grey had lived around the world. In the United States, he had been a baby-sitter, grocery sacker, carry-out boy, delivery boy for newspapers and heavy appliances, hamburger cook, yard worker, snow shoveler, car washer. He had attended schools in Japan; and at the American High School in Poitiers, France, for three years he had played on the football team. He had been an Eagle Scout and junior scout master. He said his religion was "workable."

Grey liked girls and they liked him; he was a good student; he played trombone in the high school band, danced well, sang well, knew what to do about a sick car, was six-feet-one physically. He said, after his catastrophic accident: "Mom, the best part of me is intact—my mind."

Grey was admitted to Fitzsimmons General Hospital in Denver —a fringe benefit for army families—and he stayed there for six and a half months. When they transferred him to Craig Rehabilitation Hospital in West Denver, he could make only shoulder motions and flail his arms. They fitted him with carbon dioxide-powered braces on both hands, and he was able to come home for Christmas 1963.

One day the neurosurgeon said he'd talk with Dorothy. "The neurosurgeon told me that henceforth Grey's only motion would be to move his head from side to side and grin," Mrs. Keinsley said. "If this was true, I knew Grey's life-span would be very short. But I didn't believe it."

A few weeks later, the neurosurgeon gave it to Grey—straight. Grey listened attentively and thought a minute; then he said to the doctor, "One day I will swing my legs off my bed and I will offer to bet you I am going to walk. At that time, put your money where your mouth is now."

Mrs. Keinsley saw it this way: "We have not had adequate finances to be classified as affluent, but we've had twenty years of training in frugality, and this made me astute in managing." The Keinsley mother and son got help from several sources; but all of them together didn't quite pay the medical bills.

Mother and son did draw heavily on one resource. Dorothy said, "Grey loves all life and the world. His pantheistic approach has served as a buffer against the cruelty of the world and the cruelty of man to man when adversity strikes.

"I have a strong faith that God will never give one a bigger burden than one can carry, although there have been times when I thought He punched my card twice."

Grey read Ann Sullivan's article about DMSO in *Pageant* magazine. The part about the rejuvenation of plants made him wonder: "If DMSO will do this for useless limbs on trees, what would it do for useless human limbs?" He wrote to Jacob, and his physician made the tests Jacob had required. On February 13, 1965, Jacob came to the Littleton home of the Keinsleys and swabbed Grey's neck with DMSO.

"The most dramatic change happened that first day," Dorothy told me. "Grey had had a constant pain in his right shoulder from the time of the accident, and he had learned to live with it. Late that day, Grey discovered the pain had gone. He was almost incredulous. He expected the pain to return, but it never has.

"Other improvements were gradual, as Dr. Jacob had predicted they would be. One of the welcome changes was in his thermostat; until DMSO, it fluctuated between excessive heat and cold. His body temperature became normal."

Neurosurgeons and neurologists will say that there is some spontaneous return of function for the traumatic paraplegic—but only in the first two years following the injury. If significant improvement doesn't occur within that time, it never will. There seemed to be no documented case to the contrary.

That principle is passé.

These are some of the battles as Dorothy recorded them, in Grey's war:

4/5/63   The accident. Grey was expected to die. He lived in a respirator.
2/5/64   Leaves Craig Hospital and starts classes at U. of Colorado, Denver Center.
2/13/65   Starts DMSO treatments. Shoulder pain stops.
5/1/65   Temperature sensation stabilizes.
6/1/65   Healthy color replaces pallor. Grey feels fine and smells terrible (from DMSO). He no longer is constantly tired.

Return of major functions of the body:

8/22/65   Lifted both arms over head and put on T-shirt without help.
9/12/65   Pains in left hand and wrist. First since accident.

10/17/65   Sensation to touch on right side of body starting to move below nipple line (2 to 3 inches).

10/29/65   Severe pains in right hip.

11/1/65   Sharp pains in upper left arm for several hours.

11/9/65   Severe pains in right hand and arm.

FDA banned use of DMSO

Pains subsided in a few weeks but he did not lose any of the improvements.

11/6/67   Stops wearing body brace (similar to corset to support lower back).

8/22/68   Resumes DMSO.

9/6/68   Tingling sensation deep inside neck in area of lesion.

10/7/68   Pains start again in left hand.

10/9/68   Feels heat in right hand from coffee cup—first time.

11/16/68   Moves right leg—feebly.

12/11/68   Exerts pressure shaking hands with right hand.

12/31/68   Sensation to touch on entire right side of body. It is spotty and not too clear.

1/19/69   Exerts very weak pressure with left hand.

3/5/69   Moves right thumb.

4/1/69   Raises right leg in bed.

4/13/69   He lifts his body slightly off the bed or wheelchair by using his arms locked at the elbows.

6/6/69   Grey receives his Bachelor of Arts degree in economics.

6/17/69   He moves toes on both feet—weakly.
   thru 8/12/69

10/12/69   Moves left leg—feebly.

1/1/70   He writes by hand legibly and at length.

8/17/71   Grey received his master's degree and began looking for a job, preferably in a bank.

The chronology omits mention of the many people and organizations who lent help of various sorts: The Mayfield Foundation, which supplied a hydraulic hoist (so his mother could lift him into the family car) and an electric typewriter, cab drivers who gave him a lift until the state arranged transportation to and from school, and student grants for his tuition.

The people most responsible for Grey's victory were his mother and his sister, Pamela. Pamela worked while attending school, helped her mother a great deal with household and nursing chores.

Mrs. Keinsley had to get up at five every morning and spend two hours preparing Grey for school; he required a catheter or condom to void, and even with the hydraulic lift, getting Grey into the car and into school was an arduous job. At first, Dorothy attended classes with him and made notes for him.

Grey supplemented the meager family income—from welfare, child support, and Pam's baby-sitting jobs—by grading papers and tutoring students; this brought in a cool twenty-five or thirty dollars a month; he dictated his comments and grades to his mother, who, necessarily, was his almost constant companion.

When Grey first proposed writing to Jacob, Dorothy hesitated. She was afraid that if Jacob rejected the idea, it would crush her son. She had earlier received three flat and emphatic medical opinions that her son would be completely helpless for all his days. She asked Grey: Could he take it if Dr. Jacob was negative? They sent off the letter to Portland.

In insisting that her son would find help, Dorothy Keinsley did not delight all the doctors. "One doctor bellowed at me like a bull moose in rutting season," she said. "'Don't you know your son is paralyzed?' He screamed. I explained that no one knew it as well as I."

Mrs. Keinsley said that Jacob not only did not charge for his services, but, out of his own pocket, paid the bills for the exhaustive medical examinations, which were done locally. Jacob makes a house call at the Keinsleys' whenever he is in Colorado.

When three years of supplication by himself and many others had brought no sign of relenting from the FDA, Jacob decided to resume treatments anyway. He told Grey he thought that injections into the back of the neck, in the vicinity of the scarred spinal cord, might speed up recovery; he asked if Grey was willing to accept the considerable pain of the injections and the increased odor from them. Grey agreed, but first he wanted to square it with others. He talked with his professors at the university, saying he was willing to drop out of school to save other students from the aroma. One professor said, "Grey, I want you to attend classes as usual. If worse comes to worst, there will be two people present in your classes—you and I."

The students, every single one of them, stuck with Grey, rooted for him, helped him however they could.

"In the three years that DMSO was denied him," Mrs. Keinsley said, "Grey did not progress, but neither did he lose any of the ground he had gained.

"I wish I could tell you that Grey arose from his wheelchair under his own power. This is coming. We are working toward that goal not only for Grey but for all people who are paralyzed by spinal injuries."

A specialist in orthopedic surgery and fractures has drawn up a series of exquisitely detailed reports on the nerve-by-nerve and muscle-by-muscle comeback of the patient. They probably are without parallel in medical annals.

The road back from disaster within the central nervous system is, necessarily, long and rocky. It can be also a terribly, terribly painful one.

Brian Sternberg was the world's champion pole-vaulter, and above and beyond that, a young man of high spiritual, moral and intellectual attainment, as a student at the University of Washington. Exercising on a trampoline, he leaped high, came down on the back of his neck, and lost almost all use of his arms and all muscles below his chest.

Brian's father, Harold, a successful contractor, in 1969 told me that Stanley Jacob and Brian's physician had treated him with DMSO; but Brian had given it up—it was just too painful. In bringing sensation to body areas which had been numb since the accident, DMSO had induced great pain—more than Brian was

prepared to bear. Harold Sternberg said he did—and he didn't—
want to see Brian go ahead with DMSO treatments.

"DMSO rouses pain in Brian," Harold said.

"In the sense of waking up sleeping nerves?" I asked.

"Yes," Harold Sternberg said. "The sensitivity in his legs is as
though they were being chopped up with razor blades or ground
glass."

His father said that Brian's thought processes were unim-
paired. "They're sharp—very sharp," he said. The young man had
become a ham radio operator and had made a wide acquaintance.
Many of his friends, coming upon an accident, communicated the
facts to Brian, who, in turn, relayed the information to the police.
He met a lot of people on the Citizens' Band.

At this time—seven years after his accident—Brian was losing
the use of some muscles, but he still led an exciting, if sedentary,
life. He even had romantic interests. Students at Seattle Pacific College helped take care of him. And Brian sat in his wheelchair in
the press box of the stadium and athletic pavilion for his alma
mater's main home games. He was a spark plug in the regional
Fellowship of Christian Athletes.

DMSO, applied to his skin, cleared up a pretty bad case of acne
that had embarrassed Brian. But it also brought sensation—in this
case meaning pain.

Then there was the bad sore Brian had. "This was a mean one,"
Harold said. "It was beginning to matter. We covered it with
DMSO. It took four days for the healing process to start with a
thin scab; and on the eleventh day the scab fell off, and there was
pink skin under it. They had told us you can figure a bed sore to
mean three months in the hospital and twenty-five hundred dollars. In this case, there was no hospital at all, and Dr. Jacob gave us
the DMSO."

Among the most obscene terms in medical science are—and you should excuse the expressions—"subjective," "testimonial" and "clinical impression." They rank with "uncontrolled studies" as fit only—if at all—for back fences. In medicinemanship, the purist physician can put down the doctor who says his patient had improved or been cured, with, "Sorry, Doctor, I can't credit testimonial claims." Or, "Doctor, do you have any other clinical impressions?" Or, "I assume this was a double-blind controlled study," or, if it was a double-blind, "I must say I question the adequacy of your controls."

The layman, of course, doesn't stand a chance. The physician can dismiss all the data and all the facts and end any discussion with a single question: "Sir, are you a doctor?"

One man who had been almost blind in one eye for many years told me he had made great progress with DMSO. Moreover, he demonstrated this by walking unaided in public areas and describing objects and events. His good eye was covered.

"How much credit can I put in Joe's story?" I asked the ophthalmologist.

"Not too much," he said. "Joe is looking for miracles. There's no improvement, actually. We can measure it."

"Then he really doesn't see color with his bad eye, as he claims?"

"Well, that's subjective," the doctor said. "You can't measure that objectively."

Prior to treatment with DMSO, Joe could distinguish only light and dark—not form or color. Now the man had identified for me size, shape, form, color; he could describe motion and action in considerable detail.

"I know," the eye doctor said. "I've talked to the physician who's been treating him with DMSO. But I haven't been able to check a thing so far that's changed."

Joe said, "Well, he's the doctor. But it's my vision."

And the physician who had treated him, Stanley Jacob, said, "Joe's right. I've tested it; his vision has improved."

Other blind patients have been chided by their ophthalmologists. A midwest woman wrote:

Dear Dr. Jacob:
Dad's ophthalmologist refused to acknowledge Dad's eye condition. He said there was no improvement.

Now for the facts: Dad walked from his house to the bus-line 2½ blocks, caught the bus, walked a block from the bus to the doctor's office. After the exam, he walked eight blocks to shop for a suit, then another three blocks to a shop that had recently moved —Dad had no trouble finding it or finding his way home. Dr. A.B.C. says, "Dad is such a determined man." Nuts! Dad can see.

A year ago when he started on DMSO, Dad was completely dependent on his wife, neighbors and my husband and me to take him to the store or bank, to cut his meat, to do everything. Now he takes care of all his affairs, watches TV, and is immaculate. A year ago he was messy and a constant worry to all of us.

Physicians usually say their killjoy attitudes "save the patient from false hope." Their practices often shatter all hope—true or false.

An eastern dentist, who had been under DMSO treatment given by a couple of urologists for Peyronie's disease, a painful and hard-to-treat disorder of the penis, wrote Jacob:

On February 18, one of my urologists, Dr. L., gave me injection #14 of DMSO. Palpating, he was happy to note that the plaques were practically gone.

On March 10, Dr. R., the senior member of the team, injected #15, and in the exam he said he saw the same plaques as when we started originally.

That threw me really. I got so tired and discouraged I stopped going for injections, always intending to resume but never actually doing so.

Until then I had felt fine. If I slept better I'd have been a dynamo.

With the DMSO on hand I have performed miracles on some patients—headaches, backaches. It's great for erupting wisdom teeth in young people.

The conservative majority of doctors contend that the answer to moot clinical questions is controlled studies. They feel that these experiments—especially those of a double-blind nature in which neither the patient nor the physician knows who is getting the test drug and who the placebo—will determine whether a drug is safe and efficacious.

FDA officials complained that the big trouble with DMSO lay in the lack of controlled studies. Some said all evidence had been "testimonial-type."

Actually, there have been many controlled studies with DMSO. They were conducted by well-regarded physicians, sanctioned by the FDA and run under the most rigid regulations ever proposed for a candidate drug.

In fact, it would be difficult—if not impossible—to name a medicine which has been subjected to stiffer tests for safety and efficacy than DMSO, or which has passed with higher grades.

J. Harold Brown, M.D., of Seattle, has run several double-blind tests of DMSO in cases of acute musculoskeletal troubles—strains and sprains of the neck and upper and lower back, tendinitis and bursitis. Brown is a specialist in industrial (aerospace) medicine and, in this capacity, a consultant to the federal government.

Patients were given complete physicals, eye examinations, x-rays of the injured parts and several blood tests. Their histories were taken and their degrees of tenderness, pain and limitation of motion graded. The mathematical probability of error in results was defined by what are known as chi-square tests.

In a typical series, 13 of 15 strain and sprain patients on 80 per cent DMSO had excellent responses and the other two good, as compared with none on the placebo (10 per cent DMSO), and 9 of 15 showed a good or excellent response to standard treatment. The average number of days lost from work during the first week after injury amounted to 1.2 for those on 80 per cent DMSO, 6.5 on placebo, and 4.4 on standard therapy.

In bursitis and tendinitis, 8 of 10 treated with 80 per cent DMSO had a good or excellent response, and so did all of the ten on standard therapy. None on the placebo reported benefit. The average number of days lost from work was 1.1 for the DMSO-treated, 3.1 of those on standard therapy and 6.2 on placebo.

No serious toxicity was seen.

That was one of scores of controlled studies ignored by DMSO's critics and the FDA.

I talked with Brown in his office in downtown Seattle on his "day off"—a Saturday in September 1970. Middle-aged, easygoing, he was interrupted constantly by patients who dropped in. He talked with them briefly, answered their questions, prescribed for a few, and sent each one away with a gentle pat on the back.

This is what he told me:

In 1965, a physician friend who had been using DMSO mentioned Dr. Jacob's article in *Northwest Medicine*. I had read the article, and I dismissed it as fantastic—a distortion of the truth.

Nevertheless, since my friend had success in using DMSO, I tried it.

The first patient seen had an ankle terribly swollen and so painful he couldn't bear weight on it. I swabbed DMSO on it. The swelling subsided while he was still in the office. He walked out. All this within one hour.

I decided to find out more about DMSO by becoming a clinical investigator for Merck.

I'm suspicious of all drugs. DMSO is no exception. But the longer I use it, the more enthusiastic I get. I think one of DMSO's greatest values will be in rehabilitating the injured workman.

I don't share other investigators' great enthusiasm for DMSO in the treatment of arthritis. DMSO may work well on certain arthritic conditions; anything may, including prayer. We don't have a very good scientific basis for its effectiveness in arthritis.

I tried DMSO on probably a hundred cases of arthritis, and I obtained excellent results in many. They still say it was the only thing that gave them relief, but I'm still not convinced. There are psychosomatic factors affecting beneficially and adversely all chronic diseases, including arthritis.

In acute musculoskeletal conditions, it's different. DMSO gave relief within an hour or two; with the placebo, there was none. We tried to eliminate patients susceptible to psychosomatic influences.

DMSO was taken out of the hands of clinical investigators just before a good friend of mine, Dr. Jim Goddard, became the Administrator of the FDA. He inherited the DMSO problem. I knew him to be an extremely dedicated man, a very honest man, a sincere individual—one who would do his best to straighten out the bureaucratic tangle which the clinical investigators and people felt the FDA had not solved.

The severe adverse problems occurred in animals—and with tremendously high doses. The clinical investigations had been halted. Similar problems are found in almost every drug tested on animals for toxicity if extremely high doses are used.

The DMSO ban caused much anguish among my patients. For some I could not substitute comparable therapy. I provided DMSO as long as I had a supply. There was no humane alternative.

Sometimes the Oath of Hippocrates and our personal professional ethics transcend other laws. We may be forced to decide which set of laws we must break. I would rather break the law of man than the law of God.

Following the discontinuance of treatment some patients reverted —perhaps not entirely—back to the physical situation before treatment. My phone was jammed with patients calling and asking, "When are we going to get more—when is it coming back for investigative or prescription use?"

Hardest hit were patients with chronic conditions such as the arthritics who had been benefited.

Dr. Jacob is undoubtedly one of the most unselfish, unassuming, scientifically zealous individuals that I know. And it's my opinion that someday in the future this man's contributions may be recognized sufficiently to entitle him to be considered for a Nobel prize. I said this to Dr. Goddard.

Dr. Jacob has never asked for one thing for himself. He has never made one cent out of this discovery. It has cost him a young fortune out of what is by professional standards a meager income. He has suffered emotionally; he has been castigated. He has been almost Christ-like in his ability to withstand the sticks and stones of his enemies and critics, professional, political, and lay. He has survived only because he has the support of many colleagues and of his institution.

Dr. Goddard was extremely honest and dedicated. He had no thought of personal gain. He wanted to do a good job. But he had to talk out of two sides of his mouth; one as an administrator and a bureaucrat and one as a physician.

Many doctors doing investigative work didn't know all the law— that which pertains to the interstate shipment of drugs, for instance, or the requirement for voluminous clinical records. Many clinical investigators who dealt with DMSO made similar mistakes. But they did not have the name Jacob, the prime discoverer of its therapeutic benefits, the target for the FDA.

Dr. Goddard told me, the year before he left office, that he was amenable to submission of an IND from one of the pharmaceutical houses which had been doing a considerable amount of work with DMSO. He did believe that DMSO was worthwhile, especially in short term therapy in acute muscular and skeletal problems. He said, "Look, I'm ready for it. The pharmaceutical houses aren't

219

sending applications to me. I can't go out and ask them to do it." When I proposed this to the pharmaceutical houses, they listened, but nothing was done. They said, "We are afraid. Our dealings have been with one of the other doctors in Dr. Goddard's office. If we go over his head and shoot the DMSO NDA directly to Dr. Goddard, we may lose out with the other drugs by embarrassing him. He could delay their acceptance for one reason or another."

I think the drug houses have learned to be patient with the NDA. Their very life, as a major industry in this country, depends upon their patience with bureaucracy.

Unless bureaucracy can recognize that DMSO has value, if only for the treatment of muscular or soft tissue problems, then all the scientific effort expended thus far will have been in vain.

Richard Brobyn, M.D., in his studies at the University of Pennsylvania, pre- and post-doctoral, wandered into fields he found fascinating—a great deal of experimental animal work, bacteriology, math, three years in the physical sciences, physical chemistry, along with several years as a resident in surgery. Brobyn told me the story over dinner at his home on Bainbridge Island, near Seattle.

One October night in 1964, as a young and brand-new representative of Merck Sharp & Dohme, he went to a Northwest Rheumatism Conference—a coming-out party for DMSO. Several drug houses were represented. The hall was crowded and noisy.

"It was wild," he said. "Many speakers didn't know what dose or concentration they had been using. I wondered how some reached their diagnoses. Their statements were extravagant—unbelievable."

Brobyn gave up on the meeting but later visited Rosenbaum and Jacob.

"These were honest people," he said. "I learned from them, although they too were still trying to work out dosages, concentrations, methods of administration, indications and contraindications. I approached DMSO with an open, critical—not skeptical, but critical—scientific mind."

221

Brobyn digested reports and data by those who knew most about DMSO—Jacob, Rosenbaum, Scherbel, Brown and many others. He then checked their claims against his own observations in his patients back in Pennsylvania.

"This 240-pound girl who did housework for us slipped in the bathroom and bashed the side of her head against the tub," he said. "It was a significant injury—a lot of swelling, blood seeping into tissues, a concussion. We applied sixty-odd per cent DMSO about six times that evening. The next day there was the typical local skin scaling and drying. But the swelling and ecchymosis [black and blue] were almost completely gone, and it wasn't hurting much."

Before the FDA cut off experimental treatment with DMSO, Merck doctors had treated 17,000 patients, Syntex about 7,000, Squibb about 2,000; and all the rest together might bring the total up to about 30,000. Not all were controlled studies; but the doctors and the drug houses were required to keep careful records.

Brobyn guessed that throughout the world somewhere between five and ten million people had been treated with DMSO, a great majority without any medical supervision whatsoever.

"You don't need 17,000 cases to make sense out of a study," Brobyn said. "I had 551 investigators working on DMSO. I never got to meet 300 of them, and these people never did get a distillate of what I could tell them about others' findings.

"There were guys who put thirty cc of DMSO into a tub of water, had their patients bathe in it, and claimed miraculous cures. In this concentration DMSO doesn't penetrate the skin."

Brobyn felt that DMSO would have fared much better if it had been used to treat only a single condition.

"Like thrombosed hemorrhoids," he said. "The clotted hemorrhoid is common—fifteen or twenty million Americans get it. DMSO is the ideal treatment; it reduces the pain, swelling, inflammation, discoloration, edema.

"If DMSO had started with something like this—low dose, short-term treatment—it would have been on the market in 1967."

Did Merck feel that DMSO might be less expensive and better than some of their big money-makers?

"There was some consideration of this, I think," Brobyn said. "But the data on DMSO indicated that it really wasn't that effective for many conditions. It wouldn't displace Indocin for rheumatoid arthritis. There may have been some thought that DMSO would threaten Indocin for gout and some kinds of arthritis.

"But if any company suppressed a good drug for commercial reasons, one would have to say that this was bad. I believe the majority of physicians feel this way, regardless of whether they work for themselves or industry.

"I think, however, there may be a gradual erosion, or dilution, of the professional concept—in law, in the ministry, as well as in medicine."

Brobyn said that "a pretty high percentage" of the young physicians in industry have not compromised their ideals: "I was trained to treat people. That's what I want to do. Something like seventy or eighty per cent of the junior staff during my time with Merck have returned to various phases of medicine. Their reason for leaving may be the same as mine—pure boredom with processing papers. The financial returns do not compensate for the emotional and intellectual frustrations."

Brobyn said he exposed the Vacaville prisoners to ten times the usual dose of DMSO.

"Ten times the dose," he repeated, "day after day, for three whole months. All the tests we gave the prisoners agree: there was no serious toxicity."

And if he had given the prisoners ten times the permissible dose of aspirin for three months?

He said, "You're asking me to add oranges and apples. What you want to know is: Is aspirin more toxic than DMSO? My answer is, Certainly!"

Brobyn thought for a long minute and asked, "You know who the first guinea pig was in that toxicology study—the first one to take one gram DMSO per kilogram of body weight? By mouth?"

I couldn't guess.

"Me. I took one thousandth of my own weight in DMSO. Annie," he called out to his wife, "you remember that?"

Annie's voice came from the kitchen: "Yes, I certainly do. You sure did smell!"

Brobyn: "I took it because I wouldn't expect a patient or experimental subject to do something I wouldn't do myself."

I asked what it did to him.

Brobyn said, "Nothing. And drinking a whole glass of DMSO."

Annie (from the kitchen): "He almost didn't get it down."

Brobyn: "I wouldn't say it tasted—Well, it tasted horrible. I was the first subject—in March of sixty-five."

Brobyn said that DMSO could not be compared with other drugs because it "can be given by many, many routes, and can be used to treat a multitude of conditions."

"You could take Mer-29 off the market—and perhaps they should have without delay—or Orinase—and we've got anywhere from one to five substitutes we can prescribe," he said. "You take DMSO off the market, and what substitute can we bring up? There is none. For many diseases, absolutely none."

Brobyn felt the optimal DMSO concentration for most conditions was on the order of 65 per cent. He said, "It goes through the skin rapidly and produces tolerable skin reactions."

Brobyn was both critical and tolerant of the FDA.

"The FDA has a tough job," he said. "It's very hard for them to enlist good people who know the ordinary diseases, who realize how miserable acute bursitis can be, for instance. It's amazing when you listen to someone who's been out of clinical medicine for fifteen or twenty years—it's remarkable how distorted their picture of the normal distribution of diseases has become. That's one of the problems with the FDA; the doctors get away from the treatment of people—they don't know that the relief of pain often can be terribly important.

"One shouldn't have to demonstrate to FDA doctors that a treatment alters the course of a disease—that it changes the x-ray pictures of an arthritic joint. A treatment can be highly significant if it merely relieves pain."

He thought the effect of DMSO on the eyes of test animals should have concerned doctors.

"One hundred thousand Americans then were under treatment with DMSO," he said. "Nobody thought to look at their eyes. If humans were more susceptible to DMSO than rabbits, we could have had a great tragedy."

He felt that his Vacaville studies were probably the most massive and detailed ever carried out. "They established the complete safety of DMSO," he said.

Brobyn said there were quite a few conditions for which DMSO could not be beaten; for some it was the only real treatment. He mentioned relief of the pain of arthritis and rapid and uneventful recovery following chest surgery ("If you use narcotics, the patients won't breathe as well and you'll have a lot of pneumonia"), recovery from burns, frostbite, or hemorrhoidectomy.

"Or," he added, "take a case I saw today—a little lady seventy-five years old with neuralgia which has persisted for years after her shingles cleared up," he said. "This pain can be so distressing that at times it leads to suicide. I examined her and sympathized. I put her on some analgesic agents, and I treated her for agitated depression.

"DMSO would have done her a world of good. But in the present climate, there was little I could do about that."

One year later, when I chatted with Brobyn, I asked if he thought physicians were beginning to use DMSO again. He said, "It would be a most improvident doctor who didn't have a little DMSO stashed away for conditions which couldn't be treated satisfactorily by other means."

Those who have run the most meticulous blind and double-blind and otherwise controlled human experiments are frank in saying their value is limited. They go farther—they say that a large percentage of so-called controlled studies, including those which pass the FDA, are scientifically worthless or unnecessary.

Brown told me: "There really is no true double-blind determination which will accurately assess the worth of a drug. If the preparation is of value, especially in acute conditions, those getting it will thrive. If it's no good, they won't.

"Despite all the plans and protocol and pains we took to disguise the drug and the placebo in my own double-blind studies, I had no trouble determining who got the DMSO; they were the people who went back to work in a short time.

"Furthermore, when you go through reports on ten or twelve thousand cases, you know whether a product is efficacious. You don't need one hundred of your own patients.

"The FDA has great faith in the double-blind protocol, and there is nothing for us to do but go through the ritual." Brown emphasized that controlled studies can and do serve a good purpose. "We are just overdoing it," he added. "And we are not distinguishing good from bad studies."

Brobyn told me, "Good control studies must be designed carefully and correctly, with all the variables built into them. Those in the journals—and those that pass the FDA—are not always well designed. Some which are presented with great enthusiasm show a lack of basic common sense—as bad as transplanting a human heart without so much as tissue-typing the heart and the recipient."

Neither Brown nor Brobyn felt that the best of controlled studies take the place of the good diagnostic eye.

Dr. Carl Djerassi, Professor of Chemistry at Stanford University and President of Syntex Research, once challenged FDA requirements for controlled studies. He said they were unrealistic, costly and tending to deprive the populace of safe and effective birth control.

Djerassi calculated the costs, in time and money, of producing a new contraceptive at $18,330,000 and 17.5 years. Included were such estimates as four chemists at $45,000 each a year for four years to synthesize the pill; development of animal models for testing (18 months); production of enough drug for testing (2 years); making radioactive drug for tracing (3 months); studying mechanism of action (18 months); *in vitro* and *in vivo* tests for formulation (9 months); Phase I clinical toxicology in rats (60 rats for each of 15–25 compounds) and dogs (16 times 15–25) requiring 6 to 9 months at a cost of $125,000; *or* for usual contraceptive toxicology 12,000 rats, 2,400 rabbits, 800 dogs and 5,400 primates for Lethal Dose-50 per cent, 90-day toxicological, teratological and abortifacient studies. His data were published in the September 4, 1970, issue of *Science*.

Djerassi said that while the sole purpose of a test animal is for extrapolation to the human, "the unfortunate choice by the FDA of the dog . . . had already resulted in the suspension of clinical experimentation with three contraceptive agents. Even the simple requirement for data on toxicity in the 'monkey' may be close to meaningless in the area of reproductive physiology unless careful attention is given to the choice of the monkey species."

The fetish for clinical controls contrasts strongly with the real need for research controls—experiments on organisms so exquisitely sensitive that a grain of salt in the medium, a degree of temperature, an additional hour of light, an alteration in altitude, or atmospheric pressure, an extra touch of drought or humidity, a small sound, a little more natural or artificial radiation, a bit more or less of a food element may induce a lethal or beneficial mutation, an acute or chronic disease, or sudden death.

Drs. C. F. Konzak, Robert A. Nilan and other plant geneticists at Washington State University for decades have been gathering information on the biological effects of single physical and chemical agents, and combinations of them on the stability and muta bility of genes (DNA) and other vital structures of healthy and diseased plants. Their computerized data on such life forms as

227

barley seeds and winter wheat offer scientists and philosophers a key to understanding the profound complexities in the relationships of environment to heredity. The research suggests improved ways of feeding a hungry world, preventing mutations which cause cancer and perhaps of reversing them to treat cancer.

For those who speak with piety and pride about clinical controls, a look at the more basic biological literature can be a humbling experience.

"The best controlled clinical studies ever conducted were on DMSO," Stanley Jacob said. "But I am not running controlled clinical studies, and I have no intention of doing so at this time.

"That wouldn't be fair to my patients, almost all of whom are referred to me after the failure of conventional treatment. Most of them come in great pain and disability. They expect and deserve treatment with activity. I cannot play games with cripples.

"How could one justify fooling a paraplegic who is lying there trusting the doctor to help him. I cannot bring myself to injecting saline into his neck or treating him with DMSO too weak to give him the help I know DMSO can render."

Jacob said that he uses "historical controls" for guidance. The history of medicine gives control data, he insisted.

"If some hair grows on the head of every single one of the bald men who use DMSO regularly, I would be inclined to believe what I see," he said. "If function starts to return to a quadriplegic after two years of treatment, or if a man who has been blind in one eye for fifty-five years regains some vision—well, what must one think?"

"DMSO," he said, "has met all the requirements of the FDA. But the FDA appears unmoved."

Even at this time, however, Jacob was organizing a massive controlled study on mental retardation, a field which lacked "historical controlled data."

Jacob was to learn through personal experience how difficult it often is to determine the effect of DMSO in a specific case.

He awoke in the darkness to the persistent ringing of the telephone. He heard the resident say, "Sorry, Dr. Jacob, but I don't think the ulcer case should be held until morning. There's some severe upper GI bleeding." Jacob said he'd be right over.

The luminous dial told him it was two o'clock. He rose and in the gloom dressed. Then, still in the dark because he did not want to awaken others, he walked toward the bedroom door, tripped over a toy typewriter, and went sprawling.

As he fell, Jacob's hand slid under the bedroom door, and he felt excruciating pain. He knew his finger was broken, but he didn't know how badly until he examined it in the bathroom. It was the fourth finger of the right hand—the finger he used in surgery to tie one-handed knots and to wield instruments. The distal and middle phalanges were broken and the extensor tendon was severed—a "mallet finger," such as happens when one catches a fastball on the tip of the finger. These were guesses—but expert guesses.

Jacob had a horrifying thought: supposing he couldn't operate any more?

A large lump rose on his forehead and another on his eye even as he gazed into the mirror. He swabbed both lumps with DMSO, and they went down rapidly.

His broken finger went untreated, because he would be staffing the case and wearing gloves. In 75 per cent of operations, the surgeon winds up with holes in one or both gloves—sometimes holes so small he doesn't notice them. Jacob felt it was one thing to administer DMSO to a patient who knew he was getting it, but quite another, even inadvertently, to apply it to the viscera of a patient in no position to object.

He scrubbed up and had the resident perform the operation while he stood by—just in case. In the eight or nine operations he staffed each week, he usually served as an assistant, because "the only way residents can learn surgery is to operate."

The operation—a vagotomy and pyloroplasty—stopped the bleeding and cured the patient of his duodenal ulcer.

Jacob treated his head, eye and finger with DMSO when he got home at 7 A.M. By 9 A.M., all discoloration had gone. He then went back to the hospital, confirmed his diagnosis with x-rays, and immobilized the finger for three weeks. He was lucky; in another month he was able to gown and glove again.

He was well again, and his career had been saved. But he did not know what, if any, role DMSO had played.

One does not have to examine the brand of science practiced in Nazi Germany for evidence of recklessness and the cruelty of some "controlled experiments."

The "Tuskegee Study," came to light forty years after it was initiated by the U. S. Public Health Service in Alabama. Presumably in pursuit of knowledge, the federal government's Control Cult in charge of this experiment bribed 400 black men in Alabama's Macon County to reject treatment for syphilis. This bribe consisted of free treatment for other diseases, burial expenses and fifty dollars cash. The subjects went to their graves with the dreadful disabilities of this disease without benefit of penicillin and the other anti-syphilis compounds available from the 1930's until disclosure of the facts in July 1972.

One blustery spring morning in 1970, Bob Herschler called Stanley Jacob. "We'd like you and Bev to come up to Camas and take dinner with us," Bob said. Jacob accepted at once.

It had been three and a half years since the two men had had any contact whatsoever. In October 1966, Jacob had mailed Herschler a rundown on his second meeting with Goddard in Congressman Duncan's office in Washington; Herschler mailed it back to him, unopened. Jacob called Herschler at his home; Bob's wife, Jan, said Herschler did not want to talk to him. At the Vienna symposium, Herschler had avoided Jacob; he was a lonely figure.

It was during this period Jacob, instead of taking umbrage, had Norm Kobin, the lawyer, draw up an agreement under which he and Herschler would split fifty–fifty any financial returns either should ever realize on DMSO.

At this point each had assigned his royalty rights away. Herschler, under the terms of his employment as an inventor, did as his job required—he turned all royalties over to his employer. The employer was to give him "due consideration" for each invention.

Jacob, on the other hand, had not been hired to invent anything for anybody; as a teacher, researcher and doctor, he had no contractual rights to surrender any royalties; but voluntarily, he had agreed to give all royalty rights to the University of Oregon. While Jacob did not want royalties, he did expect much of the funds to be used for research at the medical school, and particularly in the Department of Surgery. Herschler, as a partner, might then have support for himself, his family and, most important, his research, if Crown should decide to sever the strained ties with its chemist.

So on this March evening, Stanley and Beverly Jacob drove across the Columbia and up the river to Camas.

"It was like old times," Jacob told me. "The Herschlers went to the trouble of whipping up my favorite dish—spaghetti with hot sauce and hot peppers. Bob showed me his work with fish and plants."

Herschler told Jacob that he had been reluctant to disassociate.

Jacob told me, "Bob showed me a letter in which Crown gave him permission to attend the Vienna symposium; they spelled out that at this meeting he was not to be seen with me or with Dr. Leake.

"At this time there was a question as to whether the FDA was going to institute criminal action not only against me but Bob and Crown, as well. Bob said that, deep down, he was happy I was fighting back. He was fighting for his job."

By the fall of 1970, Herschler said he had been stripped of his authority, such as it had been, and his duties at Crown. I chatted with him on the telephone from Portland; from what I had heard, a visit from me could have embarrassed him in his uneasy, sterile relations with Crown. I asked him whether he would answer a few questions.

"I'll either answer or I won't," he said. He explained that he didn't mean to sound rude but at that time he didn't know how or when he wanted his story to come out. He thought, however, that what he told me would be safe to disclose by the time this book was published.

Some of the early events had become a bit vague in Herschler's memory, but he thought he first had noted DMSO's ability to penetrate plants in 1959 or 1960 and sometime later its capacity for transporting dyes and fungicides into plants.

Had he published his data? He answered, "No, I'm not allowed to."

The patents, he said, were in the name of Crown, not the University of Oregon.

"The University of Oregon, in my opinion, from a business standpoint at least, made a more definite contribution than Crown," he said. "Crown had never been interested in this until people talked about grandiose amounts of money. Then, all of a sudden, their ears picked up. But this kind of interest waned in a matter of a week or two. Nevertheless, they claim the patents. This by reason of the fact that they've gone out and gotten them."

I said I had heard that Crown had been making him uncomfortable.

"Well," he answered, "I think they're more concerned with me as a publicity focus. They've never been quite sure whether they could keep me out of the limelight if the DMSO thing really broke. I myself am not interested in publicity. I don't blame Crown for that.

"Things went as they did because we didn't really get much support—except at the medical school."

Herschler was asked, "And you both have taken a good deal of abuse?"

"It's a rough world," he answered. "We'll either come out of it all right, or we won't."

Harking back to the beginning of his involvement with DMSO, Herschler said, "I had an interest in biological chemistry, *per se*. I felt we had a number of interesting chemicals, among which was DMSO.

"When I brought the subject up, I got as much interest from Crown as if I'd suggested they extract gold from seawater. I finally got a commitment to go over to the University of Oregon Medical School or to the University of Washington and see if I could hire someone as a consultant."

He mentioned with a trace of bitterness his efforts to induce Crown to support DMSO research. On one occasion, he said, Stanford Research Institute was willing to put up $15,000 to Crown's $5,000 to determine whether DMSO would make anti-cancer drugs penetrate tumors in experimental animals.

"The nitty-gritty of this was that Crown wouldn't give the five thousand," Herschler said. "They threw up their hands.

"Anyway, Stanley finally got the animals. We put together a design for the experiments. We did our first membrane penetration studies in the dog bladder."

Herschler said he was amazed that so many people had worked with DMSO as a solvent without ever recognizing its penetrant-carrier properties.

"It didn't require a stroke of genius," he said. "Anyone with his eyes open should have seen it."

He said:

I'm not a great chemist. I'm not a great biologist. I'm just, I think, a pretty good observer.

I'd be very anxious to have my own laboratory one of these days. I expect Stanley would too. If any revenues were to come in, we might do something yet. Important as DMSO is, there might be many other interesting compounds to work with.

Industrial research doesn't appeal to me any more. I've had it. It's just fight, fight, fight.

Crown just wants to grow trees. I would like to do some good things for people.

Herschler said the only problem he had with Jacob was publicity. "I hope he'll be a little more careful when he talks to reporters now," he said. "This bureaucracy back in Washington is just waiting for an excuse to launch another attack on DMSO."

Herschler recalled Jacob's early research to keep hearts viable with supercooling.

"He was very difficult to get off the tissue-preservation project," Herschler said. "When he gets onto something, he's very hard to shake off it. Once his eyes were opened to the potential of DMSO, he certainly would have to get ninety-nine per cent of the credit for developing it."

I told Herschler Jacob gave him great credit for DMSO.

"Not in the development of it," Herschler responded. "I couldn't. My hands were tied. I sent him ideas."

When I suggested that in DMSO Crown had a tiger by the tail, Herschler said, somewhat sadly, "I'm sure they're sorry now they didn't can me in about 1958. I think if they could figure out a convenient way, they'd do it now."

He said that he felt that Crown and its lawyers knew that he could challenge their rights to royalties.

How long had Herschler been with Crown?

"It sounds horrible," he said, "but twenty-two years. I could do much better for myself somewhere else, but I can't think of a place I'd rather live than right here.

"I'm forty-seven—same as Stanley. I've been here long enough so that I have retirement rights. If I quit now, I'd get around three hundred dollars a month when I reach sixty-five—just eighteen years from now."

I said, "Sixty-five? Most of my friends are dead long before that age."

"That's the way they figure it," Herschler said. "Then they'd pay your widow all you've put into the pension plan—with two per cent interest, I believe."

I asked whether he had been questioned by Goddard and the FDA, and he said, "Oh my, yes. I have been cited and given a summons, and it cost Crown a pretty penny to get me off the hook. I got blamed for letting Stanley get loose. I was supposed to have monitored him.

"Crown has given me a bad time. They've cut off our funds for the kind of research I'm interested in." He said they had transferred those who had worked with him—all but one man. "A very good man," he said. "They may fire him too, but I think not."

In his last experiment for Crown, Herschler had put salmon and other fish in two adjoining tanks, one filled with pure water, the other with 1 per cent DMSO. The fish in the DMSO tank seemed more active than the others and perfectly healthy. (In water containing 1 per cent alcohol and any of many other commonly used compounds, the fish would have died off.) Some of the fish leaped over the barrier from the DMSO tank back into the pure water tank—and after a few weeks these fish died. The reason for the death had not been determined. But the observation could indicate that sea life adjusts to a weak DMSO concentration very well—so well, in fact, that it cannot readjust to its normal environment.

Herschler said wistfully that he hoped to resume this and many other experiments some day. "It takes money," he added. "My own needs, and my family's, are most modest. Research costs money, however."

In November 1970, the American College of Surgeons issued an astounding confession that surgeons deliberately had begun withholding life-saving care and were threatening to impose even shoddier services unless patients stopped suing for malpractice.

The college described its announcement, in a press release, as a "highly unusual" step, as indeed it was. The college traditionally had been the most responsible and forthright of all the medical organizations, especially under its more illustrious leaders. It had brought into the open such practices as ghost surgery, unnecessary operations, soaking the patient for fat referral fees, and other shameful performances; and it had taken disciplinary action to restrain the more flamboyant mercenaries in its membership. Now it was telling the public to co-operate. Or else.

This is the way the college put it.

CHICAGO, ILL.—The Regents of the American College of Surgeons feel obligated to inform the public that the rising number of lawsuits against physicians is seriously threatening the quality of surgical care and increasing its cost to patients.

Some surgeons feel compelled to treat patients under a concept which stresses avoidance of litigation rather than the application of their best clinical judgement.

Instead of attempting procedures which may cure the patient, but have a higher risk of failure and exposure to the threat of a lawsuit, some surgeons may prefer to use standard, proved, conservative methods which might bring relief to the patient, but will not cure him.

The rash of lawsuits has driven many other surgeons to still another extreme. To protect themselves against possible litigation, they are being forced to order costly tests and elaborate x-rays which under normal conditions would not be required.

To protect himself against unexpected litigation, a surgeon, like an automobile driver, must have adequate liability insurance. Because insurance companies are being required to pay out larger and larger compensation, they are finding it necessary to raise their premiums for doctors. Several insurance companies have ceased to issue professional liability insurance. In Hawaii, as well as in certain southwestern and western states, many surgeons are faced with non-renewal of their policies even though they never have been involved in any medico-legal action. This may force some surgeons to give up their practice, thereby aggravating the problem of an already deficient supply of physicians.

The Regents of the American College of Surgeons believe the problem extends beyond the profession and requires increased public awareness for its solution.

There were many causes, related and unrelated, for the mushrooming malpractice actions, not the least of which was malpractice itself. One could not brush off lightly the overworked surgeon's amputation of the wrong leg, or his leaving a sponge or scissors in the belly, or his paralyzing a patient by carelessly severing a nerve, or the doctor's forgetting that the patient could have a fatal reaction to penicillin.

If there were a common denominator governing the spate of lawsuits, it might well turn out to be money, a precious commodity dearly loved by patients and their lawyers. And by many doctors too.

The doctor's affluence—his Cadillac, his membership in the best clubs, his town house and country estate, his vacations to exotic places (often tax-deductible if some sort of meeting is staged), his expensive wife—does not tend to endear him to his patients. His collection agency doesn't help.

The doctor's fees—particularly when demanded in cash—and the prodigious levies against medical insurance policies which put him at the top of the nation's breadwinners, are not regarded as one of his lovable idiosyncrasies. Other lucrative sources of income—the pharmacy he owns or has bought into, the real estate he has amassed, the stocks and bonds he has acquired—win for him equal regard.

Some patients had come to feel that if the doctor would spend less time on his non-professional business, he might have time to make a house call for a dying child, or read enough medical literature to be current with advances that his patients are reading about in their newspapers.

With patients realizing that it is the insurance company—not the doctor—that pays, there sometimes is little reluctance on their part to initiate a lawsuit. Sympathetic jurors, equally aware of this, have a tendency to find for the plaintiff—and to find big.

Many physicians feel that the principal culprit in most malpractice suits is the patient's attorney, particularly the lawyer whose fee is contingent upon the damages he can win. Most aggrieved patients, the doctors feel, would not sue if they had to undertake by themselves the legal fees involved; lawyers willing to work for from one third to one half the judgment sometimes undermine the patient's moral sense.

Whatever the answers, lawyers, who are competitors with doctors for the top income bracket, are paying for their materialism. They too are finding malpractice insurance difficult to get and exorbitant. Their clients show them a fidelity comparable to the patient-doctor loyalty and, often, commensurate with the exorbitant legal fee demands.

Medical spokesmen had complained bitterly that the Food and Drug Administration tended to encourage patients and their lawyers to bring malpractice suits. Any doctor who violated the prescriptions approved by the FDA, specifically the package stuffers' directions, might have to explain to a jury why he had deviated from the protocol established by the super-doctors of the Food and Drug Administration.

The cards were so stacked that the many saints among doctors, as well as the sinners, often settled baseless or questionable lawsuits out of court rather than risk the public charges of incompetence (always an inspiration to other venal patients), the emotional tortures and time involved in a trial, and the unpredictable, if not hostile, attitude of a jury. There was one final bit of irony to this situation: regardless of whether the physician won or lost his case in court, or whether he permitted it to be settled out of court at the urging of his insurance company, there was a chance that his involvement, innocent or not, would make him uninsurable thenceforth.

So within a decade, malpractice insurance rates in many areas doubled and redoubled and still continued to soar.

On many counts, Dr. Stanley W. Jacob was perhaps the most vulnerable physician in the country to suits for malpractice:

1) He was a surgeon, and surgeons were the foremost target for opportunistic suits;

2) He was openly treating patients with a drug declared dangerous by the FDA super-doctors;

3) He had become the personal target for the FDA's top officials in a government-versus-citizen vendetta seldom equaled in intensity, tenacity or—so far—futility;

4) The number of patients he treated was, by any standards, far greater than optimal for a medical practice;

5) The DMSO protocol he followed was his own—the proce-

dures that a capable physician would devise as a result of extensive animal experimentation, reports by fellow doctors and his own observations on an enormous number of patients.

Jacob persisted in his practices despite friendly advice by some of his peers to go slow, despite unfriendly criticism by others and despite the extraordinary game being played by the officials, whose actions and attitudes would stand to be vindicated if some patient would only sue him for malpractice.

Dr. Morris N. Green called me from a hotel lobby on a raw, cold, rainy morning in New York. Then working at Edgewood Arsenal and living in Baltimore, he was on his way to New Jersey, to deliver two lectures on DMSO, one at Ortho Pharmaceutical Corp. in Raritan and the other at Johnson and Johnson in New Brunswick.

"I don't feel so good," he said. "I keep getting hot and cold, headaches, fatigue, that sort of thing." But he had to go. "I really have something to tell them this time; I worked hard on my talk." Besides, he needed a job—again. The Army was letting men go at Edgewood. At sixty, Morris's age made him readily expendable.

He said no when I suggested he come to our apartment. "I'm making some important arguments—very significant points," he said. "I'll go over my talk once more." He said he'd send the text of his lecture later.

A week or so later, I received a note from Baltimore. He said he'd had a coronary in the lobby of the Americana, although he hadn't known what it was, and went to Ortho and gave a two-hour lecture the next day. He had had an uncomfortable night before the lecture, but he has felt fine ever since. When his doctor saw him on Saturday, however, he sent him immediately to Sinai Hospital, where he would stay for the next three to four weeks. But he told me that the people at Ortho responded enthusiastically to his talk on the cancer therapy potential of DMSO. He was eager to explore his tumor necrotizing agent "which you remember I told you scoops out CA like a grapefruit."

On Thanksgiving Day 1970, Green wrote to Stanley Jacob that he had achieved "Step 2 recovery stage. I now walk upstairs." He called attention to papers by Scandinavians at the Histochemical Society meeting on the effect of DMSO in demonstrating dehydrogenase and in "fine structural localization of reductase and transferase in muscle."

Green said, "After January First there will be a big Reduction in Force at Edgewood and I will be surprised if I am retained. I have not heard from Ortho or Johnson and Johnson.

"I would love to continue with my grapefruit experiment in tumors. This method is a new principle of tumor chemotherapy. One uses a non-toxic method to starve or sensitize tumor DNA and then knock it out by another non-toxic method. The Green Procedure.

"The era of treating tumors with agents which are very toxic or immunosuppressive is over. In my non-toxic procedure, neither single agent does the job alone, but the combination wallops the tumor."

Morris Green left the fields of theoretical and practical cancer chemotherapy forever. Still waiting for answers to his neatly typed applications for employment—with enclosures listing the unimpressive titles he held in the nation's most prestigious universities and the more than thirty scholarly papers he had published—he died in the 1971st Year of Our Lord and the sixtieth year of Morris Green on earth. A second coronary killed him before he could recover from the first.

Shortly before Christmas—on December 22, 1970—the United States Patent Office issued Patent Number 3,549,770 for "THERAPEUTIC ADMINISTRATION OF EFFECTIVE AMOUNTS OF DIMETHYL SULFOXIDE TO HUMAN AND ANIMAL SUBJECTS." The text, embracing thirty-seven claims, covered thirty-four columns of type. The attorneys involved said it represented the broadest approval ever given to a medical advance by the U. S. Patent Office.

The patent was issued to Robert J. Herschler of Camas, Washington, and Stanley W. Jacob of Oswego, Oregon, assignors, by mesne assignments, to Crown Zellerbach Corporation, San Francisco, California, a corporation of Nevada. Another patent, under the title "RETARDING THE GROWTH OF MICRO-ORGANISMS WITH DIMETHYL SULFOXIDE," was issued simultaneously to Herschler, alone, as assignor to Crown Zellerbach; and in twenty claims it described DMSO's asserted ability as a single agent or in combination with antibiotics to control plant viruses and other industrial pests, particularly those resistant to other preparations.

Thus, with the Food and Drug Administration still banning DMSO, the Patent Office was honoring claims made for the drug by its investigators.

242

The patents were a long time in coming—more than seven years—an extraordinary delay which some said was a measure of the pressure the FDA could exert on the Patent Office.

Patent No. 3,549,770 was one of ten applied for by Herschler and Jacob back in 1963. But, by virtue of the vast sweep of pathology for which DMSO was cited, the detail of its administration, and the results achieved in numerous patients and animals set forth as examples, this was the most important of the patent applications. The other nine applications covered more specific and limited areas of use—in pain, inflammation, tissue damage, arthritis, respiratory distress, emotional troubles, infections, muscle strain and spasm, burns, skin grafts and vascular insufficiency.

The patent listed as DMSO drug forms lotions, sprays, ointments, paints, suppositories and injectable solutions. And it mentioned such methods of administration as topical, several injection routes, instillations and oral. (In the single therapy eventually permitted by the FDA, by contrast, DMSO could be used only topically, no more than 100 cc a day, for a maximum of thirty days—and only in horses, and, more precisely, non-breeding horses.)

In describing DMSO's wide spectrum as a drug, the patent preamble states that, "Unlike many other medicaments, it is useful in the treatment of apparently unrelated syndromes. The range of its activity and utility is such that it is not believed to be possible in the present state of medical knowledge in all instances to describe the activity utilizing classical medical definitions."

DMSO dosages mentioned in the patent range from 0.02 to 1.0 grams per kilogram of body weight in concentrations of from 1 per cent to 100 per cent; and the recommendations ranged from a single application to cure an occasional acute condition to virtually unlimited frequency over an indefinite period to control a chronic ailment.

The claims cited numerous clinical cases and, occasionally, animal experiments to illustrate DMSO's effects in scores of common serious clinical conditions.

The patent outlines in considerable detail the numerous forms of DMSO, and concentrations from 1 per cent to 100 per cent, diluted with water, ethanol, glycerine and other solvents, and in combination with other pharmaceuticals.

It mentions almost the entire gamut of routes of administration, and for those calling for special forms of DMSO, it tells how to compose DMSO "paints," nasal sprays, lotions, ointments (including creams and gels), suppositories and other forms. A great many salts and other chemicals are listed as ingredients which make the DMSO solutions more or less saline, or (as with glycerine) minimize skin irritation.

Part Four

"You know," Jacob said to me, "Commissioner Edwards is a very good man. We sat there in his office and talked until late. It must have been until six-thirty. He was in his shirt sleeves. He must be a hard worker."

Jacob, on questioning, said Edwards did not take back any of the things the FDA had been saying about DMSO, nor did he volunteer to undo the damage.

"He told me his hands were tied," Jacob explained.

It turned out that Jacob and Edwards didn't talk much about DMSO. Mostly, they discussed doctors and educators they knew. It was Jacob's first chat with an FDA commissioner who didn't threaten to scandalize, blacklist or imprison him. So, while he tended to like almost every human being, he was enthusiastic about Edwards.

Charles Cornell Edwards, M.D., succeeded Ley as FDA commissioner. With a broad midwest background, a flare for oratory, and long training and practice in the slickest, most up-to-date of business management methods, he brought to his office a new concept of administration and a platoon of professionals in modern management.

Edwards got his education in Colorado, topped off with a six-year surgical fellowship at the Mayo Foundation. He undertook a two-man practice in his wife's hometown, Des Moines, Iowa, whence he moved to a Washington, D.C., suburb. The AMA hired him as assistant director for medical education and hospitals; and from this job he moved over to the big management consultant firm of Booz, Allen and Hamilton of Chicago, where he became vice-president. He and his wife were regarded as well fixed financially; she was a Cowles—of the publishing family.

The commissioner was Jacob's age, dapper, smart, aggressive, and exuding the confidence of a man who had been around. He earned $36,000 a year in his government job.

Edwards could turn a neat phrase for every audience and on every occasion—as for the Academy of Pharmaceutical Sciences:

The FDA's approach to bio-availability continues to evolve. In the implementation of the recommendations of the NAS/NRC regarding the efficacy of the drugs approved by the FDA between 1938–1962, we intend to make bio-availability one of the requirements for the approval of the Abbreviated New Drug Application.

He talked to the Institute of Medicine of Chicago in such homely terms as "We can point with pride to substantial accomplishment —we are coming face-to-face with the final challenge—the current delivery system is structured in a way that tends to encourage waste—one new approach which can impact forcibly." He stood four-square for "leadership, planning and organization," for "new alternatives for coming to grips with the critical problem of increasing costs," for medical schools "providing the young physician with the tools necessary to assume community leadership responsibilities," and "meaningful programs." He was equally adamant in opposing, "writing checks with our eyes closed," and he left no doubt but that he was against chemicals which he did not name but which presented "cumulative dangers and possible connections with mutations, birth defects, cancer and other diseases."

As an expert in management, Edwards communicated a great deal—in speeches, in news releases and, occasionally, in interviews with co-operative newsmen.

Shortly after he came into office, I wrote Edwards—and called his office—to seek an interview on his attitudes toward DMSO and to ask, again, for any evidence of the drug's serious toxicity in humans. The Department of Health, Education and Welfare has a Public Information Regulation which defines the ground rules for satisfying the curiosity of the press and the public; and under this regulation, Goddard and Ley had consented to be interviewed. Edwards managed this matter neatly with a brief note: "I believe the Food and Drug Administration has acted responsibly and in the public interest, according to the new drug requirements of the law. I will see that we continue to do so. At this time, I have nothing to add to our official statement, so an interview, as you have requested, would not be a wise investment of our time."

Early in 1972, an information officer of the department, HEW, intervened on my behalf. In response to this, an FDA press agent called me, and I told him I would like to interview Edwards either in New York or Washington but, if he happened to be coming to New York, as Washington officials often did, I'd prefer to tape the interview in New York.

The HEW man called me. He said: "You know what FDA tells me? They say you are demanding that Edwards make a special trip to New York to see you."

That was ingenious management. I wrote that I would go to Washington any time that Edwards might designate. There was no answer. And that too was management.

Both Goddard and Ley had mentioned—after they left the government—that people tended to confound the job the FDA should do with the job it actually did. It seemed to be beyond the public's capability to distinguish purpose from performance. As a result, the agency gained unearned respect and escaped punishment.

The FDA deftly exploits this confusion with a steady stream of alarums, some of them "managed" by the large propaganda staff on and off the FDA premises. Some of the announcements are seasonal (banning electrically operated toys during the Yuletide) or oriented to a news event (proposing to lower the lead content of paints, following New York City's disclosure of many poisonings of children). Some of the events could be thought up by an imaginative management-minded man while dressing (poison in cosmetics, flammable wear), or in his kitchen (put iodide labels on salt and orange juice content on orange drinks, and how about the microwave or infrared oven?), or in the bathroom (label dangerous drugs or, if that's been done too often, package them so children can't open them), or in the dentist's or doctor's office (raise hell—again—about unsafe x-rays).

The FDA has protected the public in recent years from literally endless perils; it had come out fearlessly (in newpapers and on radio and TV) against such products as clacker balls, baby walkers, pacifiers, rattles, dolls, darts, variegated foreign products, imitation milks, imitation creams, Mexican pottery containing leachable lead, mercury-carrying tuna, DDT-flavored farm products, fabricated meat, fabricated poultry, fabricated seafood, fabricated cheese. It recalled 8,800,000 sodium salt forms of vitamin C pills because the salt form was not specified on the labels. It proposed that human excreta and garbage not be dumped from *new* railroad cars except at points designated by Edwards himself. (Dumping from *old* cars could be undertaken without instructions from Edwards.) Every now and then, the FDA made a list called GRAS, or foods "generally recognized as safe," although, according to the definition of GRAS, each item might be dangerous after all.

Because liquid drain cleaners containing more than 10 per cent sodium or potassium hydroxide are regarded as unsafe for children to consume, the FDA has required packaging that is hard to open. (Presumably drain cleaners of 9 per cent sodium or potassium hydroxide are GRAS.)

About thirty-eight cents of every dollar spent in retail stores goes for products regulated by the FDA—well over $240 billion a year, the FDA states. (Occasionally it gives conflicting figures.)

FDA condemnation of a product—whether capricious or warranted—can have severe economic consequences. The death from botulism of one man who ate contaminated vichyssoise bankrupted an old company called Bon Vivant; it turned out that no FDA inspector had looked in on their operation for four years preceding the tragedy.

A few cans of botulism-contaminated soup produced at the Paris, Texas, factory cost the Campbell Soup Company $10 million although no one was harmed. (The toxin produced by the bacterium Clostridium botulinum long has been an object of interest in chemical warfare; a teaspoonful or two, properly distributed, could kill everyone on earth).

The FDA gained page one publicity from the Campbell and Bon Vivant misfortunes. A couple of months later, just as the publicity had begun to wane, preliminary tests at the National Center for Disease Control in Atlanta indicated that some eight-ounce cans of Stokely-Van Camp green beans appeared positive for botulinum toxin. Again the FDA sounded the alarm, and again the agency landed on page one. This time, however, the food was okay. Edwards managed the faux pas in a speech before the National Academy of Sciences' Institute of Medicine a few weeks later: "When a food or drug issue is raised to national attention, and very few of them are not, there are naturally instant pressures to act, regardless of whether science is ready and available. This was true some months ago in the case of the contaminated vichyssoise soup. It was equally true in a more recent false alarm over botulism in green beans."

There are numerous instances in which the FDA demonstrated monumental patience and resistance to pressures—often for years after science had adduced evidence of hazards in drugs and foods under the agency's regulations. There are such examples as:

1) Sodium cyclamate's causing cancer in mice;
2) The carcinogenic effects of saccharin;

3) Brain lesions in mice injected with monosodium glutamate; and

4) The relatively free and easy use of methotrexate, the anti-cancer drug, for conditions like psoriasis—although about twenty-five deaths have been attributed to its toxicity.

It took the FDA about eight months to act on a published report indicating that pregnant women treated with the synthetic estrogen, diethylstilbesterol (DES), sometimes bore girl babies who, when they grew up, developed a rare type of vaginal cancer. DES is used to fatten beef cattle and poultry, and human meat eaters are exposed to the residue. Despite the urging of the doctors who made the discovery, Edwards delayed publishing the facts until Rep. L. H. Fountain threatened to hold hearings on them. The commissioner said he had been closely studying the situation for eight months.

A couple of weeks later, Edwards moved vigorously against the many materials containing the anti-bacterial, hexachlorophene, which was widely used in vaginal deodorants, soaps, sprays and other cleaners and cosmetics. He explained that while there was no evidence of harm to humans from normal usage of the chemical, test animals and humans using it in "abnormal" ways (presumably in excessive amounts) had shown elevated blood levels of hexachlorophene. Even medical men—or anyway some of them—thought that this time the FDA might be right, and they stopped using the antibacterial on babies. A week or two later, when twenty-two pediatric wards reported severe staphylococcus outbreaks, the FDA relented and then periodically changed the rules so that few, if anyone, could understand or obey them.

Under pressure of its numerous fiscal, political, publicity and other programs, the FDA had to ignore some troubles of individual citizens.

One such problem was the Ames case.

Jack Ames is the president and manager of the Home Federal Savings and Loan Association in Yakima, Washington. He spent a small fortune and dedicated a large part of his last twenty years keeping the breath of life in his daughter, Frances Lorraine Ames. Some of his letters had been dictated to his secretary; others had been typed by Ames himself late at night. Some of them covered six or seven pages with single-spaced type; and many of them were so graphic in describing the excruciating pain of the girl and the terrible anguish of the parents that they are now, years later, traumatic to read. A remarkable feature of all this correspondence is that each of the hundreds of communications was original; there were no slick photocopies or mimeographed enclosures to save Ames time and trouble. The only exceptions were "To-Whom-It-May-Concern" notes written by medical specialists certifying that regular DMSO treatments—before the drug was withdrawn—had not harmed Lorraine's eyes or shown any other signs of toxicity. These had been sent along to buttress the parents' piteous pleas for permission to apply DMSO to Lorraine's ailments.

When she was five years old, back in 1952, Lorraine had a series of illnesses, including measles, polio, post-polio encephalitis and mumps and then gradually a strange neurologic disorder, which at various times had been given various diagnoses, perhaps most often multiple sclerosis. She suffered recurrent high temperatures, loss of balance, impaired eyesight, loss of bladder control. She was immobilized periodically. And always there were the recurrent overwhelming pains of contractures and from other sources.

Lorraine responded fairly well but briefly to cortisone. She was given other drugs that might conceivably help her; but they were of little use. Then, in July 1964, Ames read a story about DMSO in *Life*; and, through Jacob's good offices, Lorraine's doctors got some and applied it. "DMSO was very beneficial when no other medications would help," Jack Ames later said. "It was not a cure. But it was extremely valuable in alleviating the inflammatory part of her illness and in reducing the extent of her contractures and the pain associated with them."

When the FDA in November of 1965 forbade further use of DMSO, Ames entered upon his tireless campaign to persuade the

253

FDA to let Lorraine's physicians treat her, preferably by intramuscular injection. He bombarded with heartrending appeals such FDA dignitaries as Drs. Goddard, Hodges, Sadusk and Kelsey and Mr. Kirk. He pleaded with congressmen to use their influence on his behalf—including Senators Magnuson, Jackson, Hatfield, both Longs, and a long list of Representatives, including Wyatt, Morris, Catherine May, Fountain, John Jarman and Edith Green.

Most of the congressmen took time off to inquire into the DMSO situation and to write a, usually not very encouraging, note to Ames. The FDA people also answered the letters and telegrams that Ames directed at them; but most of their responses were businesslike, impersonal, vacuous, completely negative and they ended with what seemed a mocking line: "If we can be of further assistance, please advise."

Through intervention by Catherine May, who was Ames's Congresswoman and an old family friend, Ames finally was granted an interview with Goddard; and at long last his physicians were given permission to use DMSO by skin administration on Lorraine, but on condition that regular highly complicated physical and chemical tests be run. The tests proved impossible and unacceptable to physicians and drug houses after six weeks.

Ames described his experiences and his feelings in a letter to Congressman John Jarman on May 6, 1968:

"The enclosed correspondence I am submitting is a sample of the frustrating experiences I have had with the FDA. It is one thing to administer a law and another to completely, for all practical purposes through evasive replies, ignore an individual with an obvious critical problem."

He charged that FDA officials had dodged his telephone calls. He said that DMSO had proved safe and helpful in his daughter's case, and he blamed the FDA's feeling of "vengeance" toward Jacob for its unavailability for seventeen months.

"I am certain," Ames told Jarman, "that you or any member of your committee would hate to watch, as my wife does, day in and day out our young child's (now young adult's) legs jerk with spasms, the knees cross over and pull up, the lower leg contract until it is against the back of the upper leg, the femur pull out of its hip socket, the voice diminish to a whisper and swallowing become difficult with choking on the first bite, a fairly often occurrence. The muscular control of our daughter's bodily functions, her ability to think and express herself is being encroached upon ever so relentlessly by her neurological illness."

Ames said one of Lorraine's neurologists had told him that a foreign drug capable of releasing some contractures was being evaluated by the FDA.

"My feelings would be indescribable," he said, "if such a drug had been held back in a 'bureau drawer,' so to speak, until our daughter passed on."

When I heard from Ames in September 1971, Lorraine was still clinging to life but had been in the hospital repeatedly with a high temperature and possibly either kidney trouble or septicemia.

The FDA was not accepting the blame for Lorraine Ames' difficulties or the miseries of the multitudes of others who stood to benefit from DMSO. Paul A. Pumpian, Director of the FDA's Office of Legislative and Governmental Services, put it this way (in this case, in a note to Senator Jackson on May 19, 1967):

"While the Food and Drug Administration may permit a sponsoring pharmaceutical firm to make DMSO available for clinical testing, we can do so only after receiving a proposal for such use from a drug firm willing to accept the responsibilities described in the Investigational Drug Regulations. Of course we cannot require any pharmaceutical firm to sponsor a clinical investigation, nor can we require them to make the drug available for such use." He enclosed a copy of the regulation. "The monitoring guidelines were established for patients' protection," he said.

A year earlier, M. D. Kinslow, then Director of Legislative Services, used pretty much the same statement in a note to Jackson and added this thought: "We can certainly understand Mr. Ames' deep concern about obtaining aid for his daughter; however, to lend any encouragement to the use of DMSO in this manner and for this condition would be premature as well as an interference with the doctor-patient relationship." Kinslow overlooked the fact that Lorraine had been on DMSO with good therapeutic results and no serious side effects for eighteen months.

I can't believe that there was a note of sly humor in some FDA communications. There was the line, for instance, in a note written by Dr. William J. Gyarfas of the FDA to Jack Ames, after Ames had been bombarding the FDA for years on behalf of his desperately ill daughter: "We appreciate your continued interest in the investigational new drug DMSO."

Pumpian said in a letter to Senator Jackson: "We appreciate Mr. Ames' continued interest in the investigational new drug DMSO, as well as his concern for the general area of drug testing. If we can be of further assistance, please let us know." Pumpian also pointed out in this letter that he had let Ames know that "we are still, as in the past, most willing to authorize use of DMSO for his daughter under an appropriate investigational protocol."

The American Medical Association in 1971 unveiled an ingeniously conceived insurance program, "at a time when malpractice suits are reaching epidemic proportions." The program, sponsored by the AMA, the CNA Insurance and Marsh & McLennan, Inc. (insurance brokers and consultants), was based on "peer review," a system under which members of the local medical society would screen physicians asking for memberships in the programs, help write the policies' terms, evaluate claims against doctors and aid in administration. The program would not interfere with group insurance plans operated by twenty-four state medical societies.

The AMA announcement said the program would serve to reduce the frequency of claims against doctors, alert physicians to ways of eliminating claims, resist unfounded claims, resolve legitimate claims promptly and fairly, provide doctors with long-term financial protection at fair and realistic rates, and to research alternate methods of reparation for medical injuries.

The announcement contained eye-opening statistics:

Seven to ten thousand malpractice claims were being filed each year;

one doctor in six had been sued (one in five in New York and the District of Columbia, and one in four in California);

experts calculated one in three would be charged before retirement;

the number of claims was increasing at the rate of 10 per cent a year;

the average claim had doubled—from $6,051 in 1964 to $12,768 in 1968 in New York State;

insurance rates had risen 50 to 400 per cent and more; in Utah premiums rose from $294 a year in 1967 to $3,910 in 1969, in New York to $4,100, up more than fourfold in six years, and in Los Angeles the average was $5,000;

high risk specialties—anesthesiologists, neurosurgeons and plastic surgeons—were paying from $7,000 to $12,000 a year;

doctors who had lost lawsuits were paying on renewal as much as $28,000, with a $5,000 deductible clause;

dozens of companies were dropping malpractice insurance entirely, and many others (like Lloyds of London) were retreating from large areas.

At about this time, the associated landlords of New York were proposing their own "peer review" system. Any tenant, under this plan, who felt he was being cheated by his landlord could seek redress from a committee of landlords. Physicians may find distasteful any comparison with New York landlords, who, according to public records, include some of the most morally wretched specimens ever created, and their industrial organizations. And then again, some landlords may resent being lumped with some medical organizations and some doctors.

In any event it seemed unlikely that the AMA plan would hold much appeal to either the courts or the public.

William J. Curran, Harvard Professor of Legal Medicine, in a letter to *Medical World News*, once took to task a management consultant who had advised doctors to admit a mistake and to tell the patient it was an honest error. "Patently bad legal advice," was Curran's comment. He pooh-poohed as naïve the consultant's statement that "a judge or jury may forgive an honest mistake, but no court looks kindly on the physician who needlessly harms a patient and then jeopardizes his health or appearance by concealing the fact." Curran said that confessions of error are admissible as evidence, and "courts are not in the business of forgiveness."

Professor Curran's receding hair was dark. Dr. Stanley Jacob could turn it white overnight. Jacob gave his total effort to his patients, without ever a thought to the legal aspects. Moreover, he was utterly honest with everyone.

"Have you ever been sued for malpractice?" I asked Jacob.

"Never."

"Has anyone ever threatened to sue you?"

"No," he said. "I've never been threatened by a patient or a doctor. But I have wondered if some patients haven't considered it. Theoretically, one could argue that I should do a complete physical and take a history before treatment—even though the patient had been referred to me by his or her own physician after a complete work-up."

"Why don't you do your own complete work-up?"

Jacob said, "For one thing, I don't have the facilities. And even more important, if I tried to do a complete examination of all patients—including x-ray studies and laboratory tests—it would be prohibitive in terms of time and expense. I can examine and treat with DMSO only in my laboratory. I specialize in patients who can not be helped elsewhere. If I did not accept the referring physician's work-up and insisted on doing my own, I would have to turn away four of every five patients that I now treat. I just do not have the heart to do this to people in pain or distress who can be helped only by DMSO. Those who can be treated satisfactorily by other methods are sent elsewhere."

Physicians in Portland charged between $100 and $150 for a work-up, although they gave the patients DMSO free of charge. "I don't charge my patients a penny," Jacob reminded me. "I give them everything free."

Have his treatments hurt anyone?

"If so," Jacob answered, "I am unaware of it. I have watched carefully, and I haven't noticed any unusual or serious side effects.

With most drugs one would have to cope with side effects quite frequently."

Jacob said, "We do get complaints. Not many, but some.

"For instance, I have a program for patients with nerve blindness —that is, who are blind because of a nerve defect. I have told these patients I would take them into my program only if they would have an evaluation not only by their own physician but also by an ophthalmologist before coming to us.

"My dean received an angry letter from one patient's ophthalmologist stating that we should do this examination free.

"Another doctor relayed his patient's complaint; although she was treated courteously, she thought it was very unprofessional of me to put my feet on the desk while I talked to her."

I asked: "Of the patients you treat—with the drug and many of the facilities being paid for by you personally—what percentage offer to reimburse you?"

My question made him uncomfortable. Finally he said, "Something like one in five remembers to inquire about the expenses. Most consider themselves as guinea pigs. I think that's very good —one in five being that thoughtful. Don't you?"

I thought of the cash-on-the-barrelhead fees now being commanded by doctors, with and without work-ups, of the stern notes sent out by their collection agents, of many physicians' regular hours, sumptuous homes, club memberships, expensive cars and vacations—thanks to sick and troubled people, some bankrupt by doctor and hospital bills. I said, "No."

Crown Zellerbach fired Bob Herschler at the end of November 1971. He had gone from youth to middle age in Crown's employ; and he had spent the last year and a half without a laboratory, without duties, and with eight hours a day to sit in the library contemplating the character of his employer and drawing up plans for the inevitable moment when he would be let go.

He was given nine months' pay when he was set adrift. If he could hold on to life for sixteen more years—until he would be sixty-five—he would qualify for a pension netting him a cool $300 a month.

Meanwhile?

"I've started to push ahead on my book, whose main theme covers DMSO, Crown and the poor damned researcher who is caught between," he wrote me.

I wrote to Herschler, felicitating him on now being "free as a bird," and asking him for details on this climactic event in his career.

"Yes, I am free of Crown Zellerbach Corporation and they of me," he wrote. "I was sacked after suffering through a miserable year and a half.

"I'm not 'free as a bird,' however, and not even sure that I want to be. We have just had the season's first snow of significance, some six or seven inches, and the poor 'free' birds kept us hustling just replenishing the feeders. We are blessed with a family of noisy yet beautiful blue jays that live outside our bedroom window in a cedar planting. 'Free as a bird' to them presently means cold, wet, hungry and not very happy, apparently."

Jacob told me—and Herschler confirmed it—that at least one third of all of Crown's patents in the last twenty-three years were based on Herschler's research.

"Considering everything," Herschler wrote, "it hasn't been a brilliant career—only bright, contrasting with a very dull background. With a total research staff of about 200 and a contemporary annual budget of roughly $5 million, the successful project output has been very low.

"The discovery that DMSO is a useful drug, frankly, is the only outstanding development in the 25 years Crown has supported a research department."

Herschler ascribed his own problem with Crown to three factors "and to a crew of frightened, nonproductive, noncreative, intellectual eunuchs that now, in discord, command a sinking 'research' organization," with most of their energy sales- and production-oriented. The three factors he mentioned were: 1)

261

The slowness in which DMSO moved toward commercialization in medicine and agriculture—due to government agency inexpertise; 2) Bob's association with Jacob—"I received both written and verbal warnings through the years"; and 3) equity—"my position is that a researcher takes a major risk professionally in developing and promoting a new concept—my promotions in this equity area gained me many black marks."

Herschler charged that Crown permitted him to build a biological research facility but, when specifically forbidden to conduct DMSO drug experiments, converted the space to offices and an instrument laboratory. He said that during the year of the lab's operation, he and his associates had developed a nematocide, which destroyed roundworms when used in concentrations as weak as one part per million, and potent microbe-killers—both series presumably capable of significantly increasing production of soybeans, corn and perhaps other foods for humans.

Herschler quoted one of Crown's research executives as exclaiming, "I knew it would never sell," when advised that the German distributor, Schering AG, had given up on DMSO in fear of reprisals by the FDA against its subsidiary in the United States.

"That's when I was placed on the greased-down chute," Herschler wrote.

Congressman Wyatt, who had championed DMSO, reported that the FDA had relaxed its rules, and "it appears that the persecution of DMSO has ended."

At this time scientist-friends of mine were experimenting with blood fractions which made spontaneous cancers in mice disappear overnight. They had one major problem: the mice weren't standing up well under the trauma of injections.

I got on the telephone to see if I could get a little DMSO for my friends. DMSO might dissolve and transport the anti-cancer preparation through the mouse skin and eliminate the trauma.

A supplier, called K and K, told me to try B and B, who told me I'd have to get a release from the Federal Bureau of Narcotics and Dangerous Drugs, who told me the bureau recently had been shifted from the FDA to the Department of Justice, who referred me to JO 8-5000, the telephone number of the FDA in Brooklyn. I explained my mission:

FDA This DMSO is strictly for laboratory research animals?
I This is for mice.
FDA Yeah. Laboratory research animals. Right?
I That's right.
FDA There is no impediment to the use of the material for use in laboratory research animals. Of course, if it's to be used, uh,

clinically, on animals, that's a different story. See? But from what you've described, this is simply usage in laboratory research animals. Right?

I Yes. It's clinical to this extent: These are spontaneous cancers in the mice.

FDA Spontaneous cancers, huh?

I They're not induced.

FDA I see. It might be clinical then, huh?

I Well, what do you think?

FDA But it's strictly laboratory research there. I mean, you're not treating the mouse; you're determining what it'll do in the mouse if it's used in the human. Isn't that correct?

I They seem to be clearing up these mouse cancers by injecting the stuff.

FDA Yeah.

I So it could be that they're using the DMSO to cure cancer. Would that be permissible?

FDA Then you go into another area, in which case, investigative statements would have to be obtained, you know, there would have to be a sponsor, whoever's sponsoring this; and of course the sponsor can be his own investigator, and then he would have to notify the Food and Drug Administration of his intended work. See? I mean, you know, this is another area. In other words, this would be in the area of *clinical* investigation in animals.

I If you cure the cancers, it's clinical?

FDA Well—it could be construed that way, you know.

I You can use DMSO to cause cancer, but you can't use it to cure cancer. Is that it?

FDA Well, there is no such thing as you can't use it. You can use it. The government—the regulations aren't stopping research, you know. It's just a matter of approach here. If it fits the bill in, ah, you know, the usage in—well, I'm repeating again—in laboratory research as opposed to clinical investigation in animals. And it seems to me like we have here a sort of borderline case, because here you are causing cancer and also trying to eliminate it.

I We're not causing it.

FDA As we talk here, you see, you are curing something in an animal, but the context in which the regulation is written here is that

264

then you would be using this in the animal all the time. But you're not going to be using it. You're just using it for testing in that animal. You're not going to, in other words, if it succeeds, you're not going to, let's say, take DMSO or recommend it for treatment on tumors in this particular species of mice on a commercial scale. Now, that's not your intent, is it?

There was more—much, much more. Finally, I asked where I could get DMSO if I met all the FDA's conditions. He told me to look in the yellow pages. I was back where I started—with K and K, and B and B. And I gave up.

Congressman Wyatt's optimism didn't seem justified.

While the FDA had succeeded in discouraging almost all respectable and responsible research with DMSO, it was as effective in snuffing out experiments by non-professional people as the Volstead Act was in discouraging drinking.

I once talked with a woman—let's call her Minnesota Mamie—who was a non-professional practitioner of the healing arts.

This is the way her story came out on tape:

I've used DMSO for almost everything under the sun. We cured a man who hadn't been able to have his shoes on for three years. I got him with his shoes on by using DMSO. He had gout. He also had emphysema, and the DMSO helped that greatly. We used it by mouth and by sort of a spray. But I used it all over his chest and his back and his forehead. And at nighttime just a little bit around his nose. I treated him for nine months.

I gave him about three drops to a teaspoon of water. Three times a day. Dr. Jones nearly died when I told him what I did. He had some cattle, and he had to breed a cow very quickly. The animal that he was using and the cow weren't uh—uh—compatible. So I said, "Oh, for heaven's sakes, here's the balance of the DMSO. Use it." Just kidding, more or less. But it worked fine.

A friend of mine who's a little old lady, she's got money that rolls out of her ears, but she has this sore on her leg that she couldn't get rid of. And the doctor couldn't do anything about it. And I kept yelling at her, "DMSO, DMSO, DMSO." She thought I had holes in my head, and so did the doctor. I had at this time about a quarter of a cup left, and I applied it, but I used castor oil with it. I made a mixture of castor oil and DMSO and put it on. And the sore went away.

Stanley Jacob had been told by several sources that DMSO was being widely bootlegged.

"A lot of people receiving DMSO from other than FDA-approved sources are getting a low-grade material," he said. "It scares me.

"Some veterinarians are using crude material. The FDA, however, has permitted use of high-grade DMSO, with restrictions, in horses. Veterinarians are using it in other species, as well, and this is understandable. But they're also using low-grade DMSO. A distributor told me that Syntex is supplying no more than ten per cent of what is being used by veterinarians. The other ninety per cent is bootleg."

Jacob, following a talk before the Portland Commercial Club, was told by a port authority officer the biggest product smuggled into Portland was DMSO. Most of it came from Japan.

A pint of DMSO, even contaminated industrial grade, brought twenty dollars and up, although the legitimate price was still as little as thirty-five cents a pint, in thirty-five-gallon-drum lots. With purification to reagent grade—that is, about 99.5 per cent pure, or good enough to be used in a chemical lab—DMSO sold to industry for anywhere from fifteen to thirty-five dollars a gallon, depending on the avarice of the seller and gullibility of the buyer. Crown sold spectral, or medical, grade DMSO, the purest of all, for $1.25 a pint to Syntex, which then diluted it with 10 per cent water and sold it to veterinarians for $10.85 a pint.

Who—or what—was the FDA, the *bête noire* of Stanley Jacob and DMSO? It was an agency possibly unique in the history of government—any and all government. It was as incredible in its way as Stanley Jacob was in his—or DMSO in its.

It has been criticized bitterly by many familiar with its operations—aggrieved individuals, a large part of the scientific, medical and popular press, Congressmen, commissions and committees appointed to investigate the agency, and the highest officers of the bureau itself.

Ley told the New York *Times* after he left the FDA:

"The thing that bugs me is that people think the FDA is protecting them—it isn't. What the FDA is doing and what people think it's doing are as different as night and day."

In May 1969, Ley had appointed a "Study Group on FDA Consumer Protection Objectives and Program" which later became known as the Kinslow Committee because the chairman was Maurice D. Kinslow, who headed up the FDA's Baltimore office. The members numbered seven, with three being doctors and Kinslow and three others being "lay." All were officials of the FDA.

The Kinslow Committee in eleven weeks put together a forty-six-page report which recommended drastic changes in the FDA organization and services. While the report was regarded as a ploy to induce Congress and the Administration to pour more money into the FDA, it made it clear that the FDA was not doing the job that should be done to regulate the more than 60,000 food, drug and cosmetic firms with annual sales of more than $130 billion.

The report indicated the FDA was neither informing consumers nor enlisting their help as it should. It said the FDA was failing to curb lies in advertising, limit filth and other contaminants in food, work with allied agencies, check on the safety and efficacy of drugs, work closely with scientists, doctors and industries, and investigate hazardous products. The agency lacked adequately trained scientists, it said.

The Kinslow report was one of about a dozen critiques of the FDA produced at about this time. And it was one of the very few which showed some sympathy for the FDA. Nevertheless, the careful reader had no difficulty detecting that all was not well with the FDA. The FDA itself was saying so.

The FDA and some of its officers have been accused of lying, cheating, police state tactics, bribe taking, medical quackery, atrocious scientific judgment, being soft on narcotics, censorship, blacklisting, blackmailing, conspiring with Internal Revenue Service and other federal agencies to "get" the critics, driving small drug houses into bankruptcy, pandering to major drug houses, boondoggling, inflicting needless discomfort and death on sick people, harassment, intimidation and numerous other sins.

The recent history of the FDA has been reviewed critically in *The Dictocrats, Our Unelected Rulers*, a free-swinging exposé by Omar V. Garrison, and *The Chemical Feast*, by James S. Turner, a detailed, documented report assembled by Ralph Nader's Study Group.

One other official report gave a rather clear picture of the agency. Six prominent men in the fields of science, medicine and education, comprised the FDA Ad Hoc Science Advisory Committee, which was to "review and evaluate the total scientific effort of the FDA and to advise the Commissioner on aspects of

FDA's science activities that, in its judgement, warrant improvement."

That committee was set up by the commissioner, who was not known to flagellate himself and his associates. The committeemen were not trained and tough investigators but men of culture and professional standing—the report was remarkably candid. The members were Marion W. Anders, D.V.M., Ph.D., Associate Professor of Pharmacology, University of Minnesota; Berwin A. Cole, Ph.D., Deputy Associate Commissioner for Science, FDA (Staff Director); J. Richard Crout, M.D., Professor of Pharmacology and Medicine, Michigan State University College of Human Medicine; Willard A. Krehl, Ph.D., M.D., Professor of Preventive Medicine, Jefferson Medical College; Roy E. Ritts, Jr., M.D., Professor of Microbiology and Immunology, Mayo Graduate School of Medicine, University of Minnesota (Chairman); and Lauren A. Woods, Ph.D., M.D., Vice-president for Health Services, Virginia Commonwealth University.

The Ritts Committee, as it was called, made it clear that the FDA was not all bad—nor all good. "Thus one can find in the FDA certain laboratories with advanced technology, good morale, and high productivity which give every impression of being first-rate by the most rigorous standards," the report began. Having demonstrated fairness, the report continued: "On the other hand, one can also find laboratories so poorly managed that scientists seem unable to describe their work coherently or produce interpretable data books containing their findings."

The report, in fifty-six pages, single-spaced, listed as among the impressions recorded during one year of study:

In many FDA laboratories, the general scene is not charged with any sense of excitement or even great industry . . . the FDA has long favored the compliance branches over the scientific branches . . . the FDA has not engaged in adequate central planning; planning often failed to include opinions of scientists . . . some regulatory decisions are as defined by law, even though they may not be consonant with scientific data or opinion . . . because of erratic shifts in planning, administrative reorganizations, and new crises, scientists often must suspend or abandon ongoing work in favor of new projects . . . arbitrary administrative rulings on scientific activities are frequently made by non-scientists . . . certain scientists, instead of carrying out assignments, pursue research in line with their own interests or what they think is best for the agency, and management and central planning are so bad that self-assignments are hard to detect or correct . . . frustrated scientists take their incomplete or preliminary finding directly to the public . . . the scientific environment is encumbered with a curious aura of secrecy, an atmosphere of non-communicativeness between scientists within the agency and in universities and industry, commonly explained away as protecting trade secrets or lack of understanding of FDA problems by outside scientists.

The committee even hinted broadly at perilous hanky-panky jeopardizing the nation's drug and food supplies, when it said, "The Committee is in no way persuaded that the scientific basis for regulatory decision-making should be modified by consideration of economic or political factors."

Almost every scientist interviewed by the committee acknowledged that managerial and communications problems were "long-standing and widespread," according to the report.

Considering the punishments meted out by the FDA, one comment carries a particular poignancy: "The Committee was disturbed to discover that the FDA did not have a systematized record keeping system for its laboratory work. There was no evidence that laboratory data were being recorded in such a way as to be secure from misplacement or alteration, or to permit ready retrieval . . . The Committee strongly recommends that the Commissioner remedy this situation immediately."

The committee found that some of the FDA councils of outside scientists had not been used at all, that others were never told what to do.

The committee found that "serious deficiencies exist at all

levels" of the contracts for research (amounting to more than $6,000,000 a year) which the FDA farmed out to scientific organizations. It found the FDA guilty of bad or negligible performance in contract planning, setting priorities, soliciting bids, reviewing contract proposals, supervising research activities, maintaining a budget, appointing project managers, and in not permitting the scientists to report research.

The committee concluded that FDA District Offices are operated as "the compliance arm of the FDA" and that the scientists and their laboratories are oriented toward police work —surveillance and analytical procedures. As a result, the selection of food and drug samples for testing is sketchy and the procedures antiquated and cumbersome, the productivity per scientist low, with a preponderance of senior scientists (and dearth of technicians) who do menial work and inferior scientists who work for the relatively low pay of the FDA and tolerate restrictions against publishing research results.

One of the dangers of the FDA field setup is posed by the drugs added to animal feeds which humans ingest in meat and poultry. The widely differing estimates of drug residues in meat and poultry, the committee stated, indicate that "there may exist a situation of possible danger to the public and potential embarrassment to the government."

The committee expressed trepidation at the prospect of the FDA's announced intention of expanding its jurisdiction over foods—adding to its present badly done job of monitoring them for contaminants the additional task of passing on their nutritional qualities.

The report said, "The Committee was dismayed to learn that the FDA does not have accurate information at any point in time on the identity and amount manufactured of all drug preparations, both ethical and proprietary, currently on the market in this country." It found fault with the FDA's inadequacies in statistics and in epidemiology.

The report said the processing of applications for the testing and introduction of new drugs "is slow and erratic, demands for data may be scientifically unjustified, some reviewing officers make rather rigid and arbitrary decisions while others have trouble making decisions at all, and interpretations of policy vary from reviewing officer to officer."

The report noted charges that university investigators faced unreasonable requests which hamper research, that applications were often poorly documented, that obfuscation was frequent, and that many studies were scientifically poor. "These complaints seem to go beyond the expected grumblings of the regulated, and their persistence through the years implies the presence of chronic unsolved problems," the report stated.

The committee, commenting on the unfavorable reputation of the FDA scientists, attributed it to the belief that the safest course for the medical officer to follow is to be negative, since he will then stay out of trouble. It added, "The toll is indirect but real: difficulties in recruiting top-flight scientists into the Bureau of Drugs, diminished credibility with physicians in practice, and a low level of respect among university and industry scientists." It said the FDA medical officer all too often had "neither research experience nor prestige among his scientific peers; nor are his judgements viewed by his fellow scientists as scientifically sound."

The report described handwritten documents, typewritten communications days and weeks behind schedule, crowded offices, desks in waiting rooms, the lack of training programs. It pointed out that some studies showed 25 per cent of drugs then marketed were substandard.

The committee said, in an embarrassed sort of way, that the AOAC (the Association of Official Analytical Chemists) was the beneficiary of an affectionate financial and footsie-type relationship with the FDA. The AOAC is an independent scientific society of the United States and Canada whose principal role is sponsoring the development and testing of methods for analyzing pesticides, food additives, drugs, animal feeds, cosmetics, liquors, beverages, fertilizers, hazardous household products, air and water pollutants, and the like. The facts that the FDA puts a lot of money into the AOAC, that most of the AOAC's associate referees (298 of the 585) were FDA employees, and that the relationship could suggest financial advantages to both the FDA and the AOAC people occurred to the committee. With restraint, the report did not carry the ugly words graft or bribe or even moonlighting. The report did say, however, that:

As in issues of conflict of interest, where the appearance can be as damaging as the actual guilt, there are facets of the AOAC-FDA relationship which in the hands of the poorly motivated could embarrass FDA. As examples, certain FDA employes whose titles, grades and job descriptions indicate otherwise actually spent significant portions of their official working time on AOAC business, in the capacity of AOAC officials; at times one can be easily confused as to when they operate as AOAC officials and when as FDA employes.

It mentioned that the FDA gave the AOAC space, supplies and facilities; but the AOAC did use a non-FDA address, "even though the residence of the AOAC in FDA is common knowledge," as the committee put it. The committee added that "these facts give the *appearance* of subterfuge and an interlocking directorate."

The Ritts Committee report may have clarified one phenomenon: Despite the FDA's numerous nominal house cleanings, nothing really changed. The Ritts Committee said:

The recent reorganization was but the latest in a series of such activities in recent years, each usually accompanied by an infusion of new management at the highest levels. The Committee detects that this has sometimes in the past contributed to poor morale. Furthermore, there appears to have engendered an attitude on the part of some that nothing changes very much at mid- and lower levels in spite of such management changes at the top. This view is supported by the observations that the middle management of science of the FDA has been very stable over the years. After a reorganization, the same names are seen, but in different capacities.

A week or so after the release of the Ritts Committee report, Billy Goodrich resigned.

Jacob paid a high price, in many currencies, for his DMSO research. In terms of money, Ed Rosenbaum couldn't understand how Jacob could be so free with it.

"He's more than broke," Rosenbaum told me. "He's in debt—I wouldn't pretend to know how deep. He's had to liquidate whatever stock he has owned. Everything he has is mortgaged.

"And still, whenever a friend needs help, Stanley will give him whatever liquid cash he has. Just recently, friends asked him for a few thousand dollars; he borrowed the money to give to them."

Would his friends remember to repay Jacob?

"I hope so," Rosenbaum said. "But that wouldn't make much difference to Stan. He probably has complete faith in those who borrow, because he himself is a man of absolute integrity. He's one of the few who wouldn't have to sign a contract."

In more than twenty years of practice as a physician and surgeon, Jacob had never collected a dime from any patient. Whether this was the cause or effect of his poverty was conjectural. How could he do it and get away with it?

Jacob's annual income is in the neighborhood of $35,000 before taxes—a salary of $25,000, an additional $1,000 as a colonel in the U. S. Army Reserve; and about $9,000 in royalties from two editions of his textbook *Structure and Function in Man*.

About one half of the surgeons at the medical school have a private practice downtown, and they earn from this anywhere from $5,000 to more than $50,000 a year. Jacob spends all his spare time on research. The medical school collects the fees for surgery performed by him and other faculty members in its hospital.

The Jacob home is a ramshackle frame house in a middle-class section on the outskirts of Portland. Its market value is about $20,000; and it carries the biggest mortgage obtainable. Jacob borrows to buy a second-hand car (a four-year-old Rambler at the moment), and he makes monthly payments on it, until it is ready to expire from its infirmities, when he turns it in on another used, and sometimes vintage, vehicle. He knows little about automobiles except how to drive them, and he has no intention of learning more, because he is too busy with more important things.

Except for a jacket or slacks which a friend might give him, Jacob's clothes are in the lower price range; he wears them well . . . and long. He takes advantage of his Army Reserve duty to stock up on six-dollar shoes and other GI wear.

He combines professional travel, which is paid for, with his DMSO interests (treating patients, talking to Congressmen and bureaucrats), for which he himself must foot the bill.

His wife buys margarine instead of butter, and when Jacob eats alone, he goes to a hamburger stand. His entire estate is in cheap life insurance.

In eight years, Jacob had put about $75,000 of his own money —cash and credit—into his research with DMSO. How did he amass such a large amount?

"I borrowed it," he told me.

Jacob was not the only one who put out to develop DMSO. The University of Oregon granted about $100,000—or $10,000 over and above what it had collected in royalties—to DMSO research. Crown Zellerbach put another million dollars or so into it—and most of it for patent protection around the world. And assorted drug houses and people had sunk almost $20 million into DMSO—Merck, Syntex and Squibb a few million each, and additional millions from American Home Products, Geigy, Schering Corp. of the United States and Schering AG of Germany.

Of all the investors, however, only Jacob stood to get nothing but satisfaction out of the gamble on DMSO.

DMSO cost Jacob some of the joys of family life.

When Stanley and Beverly married, each had had a son by a prior marriage, and together they had two more sons. He was almost forty years old and well settled in his research, teaching and medical career. She was twenty-three and with a background of office work; she was lighthearted, often bubbling over with laughter.

Whereas Stanley had had the material and emotional protection of a loving family, when Beverly was about three years old her parents divorced, and she and her two older sisters grew up early.

Beverly thought that her marriage to Stanley might have lasted, had it not been for DMSO. As it was, she became a disillusioned partner in a *ménage à trois*—her husband, DMSO, and lastly, herself. So they agreed to separate—not at once, not in anger, but amicably and at their mutual convenience.

Although he was a superb physician, surgeon, scientist and educator, Jacob was not one to putter around the house.

"I taught Stanley just the other day to change a light bulb," Beverly said. "He went up the ladder, reached over the top of the shade and changed the bulb. When he came down he was so proud! He said, 'Kid, you know that's the first bulb I ever changed.'"

Beverly said—and others agree—that Jacob can be the despair of a gourmet cook. "His favorite dish is spaghetti with a complicated sauce full of red-hot chili peppers. If he can't have that, he'd like hamburgers and hot dogs smothered in Tabasco. Then he drinks cream soda to put out the fire."

Bev said that Stanley was "very protective" toward Marilyn, his divorced wife. "He works with her every day so that he can keep control of her medication," she said. "He takes her to dinner when he can get away. Their son, Stephen, visits her regularly—always on Sunday and at least twice a week when he's back from college. Marilyn is better off now than at any other time since she first became ill."

Beverly gave these insights into Jacob's character:

I don't know that he is terribly handsome. But women treat him like he's God—I think because he is so kind. Women who make a fuss over him make him feel just great; and that's the way men should feel.

He loves children more than any father I've ever seen. He dotes on them. He has never raised his hand to them, not even his voice.

Stan rescues stray dogs and cats—and stray anythings. He has brought home one patient after another, and a lot of them he couldn't even remember their names. Some couldn't afford a hotel room. I've helped bathe them, and pack them up and downstairs, and feed them. Stan treats them medically, and if they have urgent problems, he runs home from work to make sure everything's all right.

Grandpa works for the government. In 1958, he went into a field and got dust in his shoe, and this resulted in a radiation burn. Three other people went into the field with him, and two of them are dead. Another fellow had a burn all over his face. Grandpa's foot looked bad—he had only one layer of flesh over the bone. It was all purple and painful for many years. He'd wrap it and soak it, and he limped on it.

When Grandpa was up to see us, Stan said, "Well, let me take a look at that foot." He looked at it and said, "Why don't we just put a little DMSO on it?"

Grandpa, of course, was willing, and when he left there had been a remarkable improvement. Stan gave him some DMSO, and he told Grandpa to apply it every day.

We didn't see Grandpa for six months. When he came back, he said, "Stan, I want you to see my foot." He took off his shoe and sock. The layers of skin and tissue had built up. The purple had disappeared pretty much.

He had lost a good deal of vision also. But with this DMSO on his foot every day, he began to get his sight back. You'd never know he'd had a radiation burn.

Some people, when they moved, left a litter of four little puppies behind. Stan heard them whimper, found them in the deserted yard. It was raining, and the puppies were cold. Stan took them home, shivering. They had pneumonia. He gave them shots, and we fed them with a medicine dropper. He kept calling me every hour from the medical school to find out how they were doing. If they hadn't had the very best doctor in town they never would have made it. Stan stayed up nights with those puppies; he put his whole heart and art into saving them.

I asked if it bothered her to have her husband spend his talents on puppies and non-paying patients rather than on patients who would pay high fees for his outstanding skills. Beverly said she was satisfied.

"I never want for anything," she assured me. "When I ask for something, I may not get it that day, but he'll make sure that I have it. I haven't asked for furniture or anything expensive because I don't want to put him in a financial fix. But he somehow provides everything I ask for. I may have to wait a week or two, but when he delivers it, he acts so nonchalant. He doesn't want to be thanked; he says, 'Oh, that's nothing, Kid.' "

Jacob got loans from the Teachers' Credit Union, Portland banks and some from out-of-town lending institutions; and these latter were easiest of all to borrow from.

"These small lending institutions advertise," he told me. "You find their ads even in paramedical publications. They save time and trouble; and you just write a letter and say, 'I'd like to borrow $5,000.' In a few days, you get a form from them. You write your name, address and where you work. You don't have to fill out a financial statement or even give references.

"Then in two weeks they send your check. It's called executive credit; it's for executive-type people."

What interest do executive-type people pay for executive loans?

"You know, that's a very good question," he said. "I didn't realize how much I was paying until the full-disclosure law came into effect. I was amazed that this kind of loan was costing me twenty-four per cent."

At the Teachers' Credit Union the interest rate was a very reasonable 8 per cent. Some other loans called for 17 per cent.

Marilyn Jacob is Stanley's first wife—and one of his two present secretaries.

Often when her name came up, Stanley would say, "Marilyn is a beautiful woman." This was true. She was sensitive—a fragile leaf fluttering in a wintry wind. Behind her dark eyes were the torments which pills could not dispel, the agonies of a desperate effort to cope with a harsh world.

"Marilyn is my right arm," Stanley would say. She lived for him, worked for him, prayed for him. There was a weariness in the angles of her face, in the darkness beneath her eyes, even in the shy smile that cast its light about her; these were medals awarded for her gallant dedication to the man she loved.

"I worry so much about Stan," she said. "He has so many great pressures upon him—his debts, the FDA, DMSO, his profession. When I see him being pressed and hurt, I feel myself starting to go to pieces again.

"I've got to help him. And I've got to help myself too in ways that nobody else can help me."

Marilyn Peters and Stanley Jacob met in 1946. She was nineteen and a secretary for the Columbus Tuberculosis Society and he was twenty-one and an extern—a medical student beginning to make the rounds of the wards with staff officers, residents and interns—at the teaching hospitals of the Ohio State University Medical School.

"Sometimes he would walk to the bus with me," Marilyn reminisced. "Then one evening he asked me for a date. We married two years later, and we went to Boston.

"All his patients just adored Stanley. He introduced me to them. I knew everybody in the hospital—those who worked in the boiler room, the secretaries, the staff."

In 1951 Stephen was born, and two months later Marilyn was stricken with *postpartum tristesse,* that melancholy mood of unknown etiology which overtakes many women after childbirth, often to dissipate with the passage of time, occasionally—as in Marilyn's case—to linger indefinitely.

Marilyn was returned to Columbus—to St. Francis' Hospital, in which she had trained as a nurse—to recover in a familiar environment among old friends and her family.

"I didn't know who I was or where I was," she said. "I couldn't recognize my relatives."

Then one day a nurse stopped her in the hall, took Marilyn's head firmly in her two hands and said, "Now, look straight into my eyes. Have you ever seen me before?"

"I looked at her face for a long time," Marilyn told me. "Finally I recognized her as having been in nursing school with me. We went into a room and talked; and all of a sudden, almost instantly, I became well again."

A little more than a year after entering the hospital Marilyn left it—to rejoin her husband and son in Japan.

When Jacob, an officer in the Army Medical Corps Reserve, was called up during the Korean conflict, he had asked for front-line duty, but the Army kept him busy in an Osaka hospital until after the war had ended.

Marilyn found happiness in Japan . . . until the depression set in again. Then it was back to the hospital—this time to Walter Reed. It was back to electric shock treatments, and insulin shock, and whatever other inadequate therapy medicine offered. And from then on—for almost an entire decade—it was pretty much a matter of one hospital after another.

Stanley Jacob never gave up. With each new commitment, he did what he could for Marilyn's release—he worked and waited, hopefully, patiently, for the day when the fine fabric of her over-taxed nervous system would repair itself and she could return home. He dug into the literature and consulted specialists and found there was no easy way, nor any sure way at all to rescue Marilyn.

The consensus among the psychiatrists was: Divorce might help. For her own sake, for the well-being of their child, for her husband's need to pursue his profession and the demands of everyday living, there was no alternative but to relieve Marilyn of the anxieties and obligation of her role as wife and mother. The unanimity in this opinion left no room for debate.

So when Marilyn again was out of the hospital, they divorced and he found her a small, easily maintained apartment. From a distance he and their son watched over her.

Within weeks of being rid of family responsibilities Marilyn began to improve. Her small apartment posed no problems, and, with only herself to please, shopping and cooking lost their terrors.

Then she noticed a recurrence of a few of the old symptoms, and she was terrified.

"I found myself staying at home," she said. "I was taking a lot of pills. I began to realize I was going downhill."

Jacob asked his professional friends what should be done. Again there was agreement: Try occupational therapy.

Marilyn sought jobs. And she got them.

"But I was too afraid to report for work," she told me. A large department store hired her twice. And twice she didn't show up.

Then, when things looked blackest, Stanley hired her.

"You know," she told me, "I really don't think I could work for anyone else but Stan. It puts me in a bind. But that's the way it is."

Marilyn makes out Jacob's schedule for interviews and for his numerous other obligations—in the lab, in surgery, in the classroom or lecture room. She tries to fit into his routine the visitors with casual or urgent missions. She answers the telephones, which ring one at a time, or two at a time, but constantly. Most of the calls, local and long-distance, are from people who want DMSO treatment for an enormous assortment of ailments. She tells them what to do—first of all, have their referring physicians send the diagnosis and history and indicate what treatments have been tried. Jacob shields her as best he can from dilemmas and deviations in routine.

In a hurried world, Marilyn's sweetness, patience and understanding are a refreshing departure from the usual business conversations. She knows about troubles. She's had them.

"Ever since I went to work for Stan, a lot of things have been going for me," she said. "It's hard for others to know what happiness there is in just being able to walk down the street on one's own."

And now when Marilyn's door was locked, she was the one who locked it.

Once when she learned that Jacob was particularly hard pressed, she withdrew her life's savings—almost $5,000 she had accumulated from the alimony and gifts from Jacob, gifts from her family, her modest pay—and she begged Jacob to accept a bank check for that amount.

Jacob agreed to a loan. He could think of no other way out of the dilemma.

Except—and this occurred to him later—maybe Uncle Morris.

Uncle Morris was a pleasant, dark-eyed man with a soft voice and loud shirt and strong cigar. He was in his late fifties and a little on the heavy side.

Morris was the brother of Abe Jacob, who was Stanley Jacob's father. Morris's and Abe's mother was from Baghdad and was related to the Sassoons and Khadouris, who became the merchant princes of the East. Their father was from Persia and an orphan. Abe and Morris were raised in Atlantic City.

When they were young, Abe used to wheel Morris in a baby buggy along the boardwalk, where their parents had a business, opposite the Steel Pier. The family—four boys and four girls —were good students, and they lived comfortably, all but a younger girl who was killed by an automobile on her way to kindergarten.

Abe helped raise Morris, and when the two grew up they operated a retail store which handled works of art and fine fabrics. Abe, the connoisseur, met Belle in Philadelphia, and when they were seventeen they married and in due course begat Rita, Stanley and Bobby (who later died). Belle was a regal lady of great dignity and charm.

Abe was like Stanley—soft-spoken, gentle, scholarly. He spoke every Arabic dialect, and he had a sixth sense which enabled him to make phenomenal predictions of events to come.

"Everybody just had to fall in love with my brother Abe," Morris said.

His father's urging was the reason why Stanley went into medicine, and Bob's kidney disease caused him to go into transplant research in the 1940's, although the scanty evidence indicated that organs never could be transplanted in a practical way. Then Stanley and Dr. Lester Persky at Beth Israel, a Harvard teaching hospital, in 1949 dosed dogs with cortisone and transplanted kidneys to them. Their report, the first on cortisone's role in kidney transplants in the American literature, appeared in Proceedings of the Society for Experimental Biology and Medicine in 1951.

Bobby was the first person ever to try DMSO for gout—and it banished his pain promptly and completely. But neither DMSO nor any other drug could keep him alive. So this bright and beloved young man died in 1965.

Uncle Morris explained Stanley's lack of business instincts:

"He is dedicated to scholarly, scientific, humanistic pursuits. He is a giver—not a taker. So anybody can take the shirt off his back.

"Stanley is a believer. He will believe anyone. He is not and can not be a merchant. And for that we love him."

I recited a litany of Stanley's financial indiscretions. "And almost every time he failed," I said, "it was Uncle Morris who bailed him out."

Morris said, "So it's only money. He is doing something that will benefit the whole world."

Morris said Stanley was like his father.

In 1937, Abe Jacob moved his family from Atlantic City to Youngstown, Ohio, where he ran a children's wear store. "For the benefit of people who couldn't pay," Morris said. "He had many, many non-paying customers. Everything left over on Christmas Eve went to one of the orphanages in Youngstown. Abe was Jewish, but he had the Christmas spirit."

Abe was an ardent Republican. "He even bet fifty dollars that Alf Landon would carry fifteen states," Morris said. "Before the election Abe would say, 'Even a dog could carry fifteen states.' "

Stanley's mother recalled how, on the night of the election, even when there no longer was any doubt, and the announcers were saying, "As Maine goes, so goes Vermont," Stanley went to bed crying for Dad and the fifty dollars. "Even then, his dad didn't give up," Belle related. "Trying to cheer Stanley up, Abe said, 'Wait 'til the farm vote comes in.'"

Morris said his brother Abe "was born with a veil on his face—he felt he could foretell the future."

There is nothing about Stanley Jacob's behavior or about his thinking that would fit any dictionary definition of "mystic," but he had this one experience:

My father used to tell me I was destined to do something good for mankind. This was my chosen field—this was what God intended me to do, he said.

My father died July 1, 1959. About eighteen days before he died, he telephoned me in Boston. I had finished my residency, and I was instructor in surgery at Harvard Medical School.

Dad asked me when was I coming to see him. I said that I was going to drive out to Oregon and I would be through Detroit on July 10. He said, "Son, I wish you'd come out before then. I really want to see you. I want to talk to you."

I said, "Dad, this is silly. I can't afford it. It's just a question of ten days. I want to see you too, but I just can't come. I've got all of these things to get ready. I've got to get my furniture packed and finish up at the hospital."

He said once more, "But I really wish you'd come. You know, I had the craziest dream last night."

I said, "Dad, you're always having dreams."

He said, "No, this was different. I dreamed that you went to Portland, Oregon, and you were experimenting with wood rot."

I asked, "What do you mean—wood rot?"

He said, "I don't know. It looked like it was dry rot—like under ships. You found a wonderful chemical. I could see people all over the world with their hands out, asking for this chemical. When you get to Portland, get hold of some wood rot and see if there's any-thing valuable in it."

Well, two weeks later—on July 1—he died. I didn't get to Detroit on a plane until about six o'clock in the evening. Uncle Morris, Mother, Mother's sister from Philadelphia, and the family were sitting in the living room.

My father had gotten up that morning to take the bus to work. He mentioned to my mother that he had a little pain in his chest. He started to walk to the bus, but he came back to the house, and he said to Aunt Janet, "I have a terrible pain in my chest."

He went to the phone and tried to call a doctor or an ambulance or someone to help him. The telephone exchange—a university exchange—was overloaded, and he couldn't get a dial tone. Aunt Janet said she remembered him saying, "It wasn't meant to be."

And he just sat down and died.

When I got there that evening, I thought my mother was taking it pretty well. She said to my aunt Dot, "I feel faint. I think I'll go upstairs and lie down." Aunt Dot went up to accompany her. Then she called to me, "Stanley, come up. Something has happened to your mother."

I went upstairs. My mother was lying on the bed. She was death warmed over. I sat down beside her and put my fingers on her wrist. She did not have a pulse.

I was frightened. I thought to myself, "My God, she's had a heart attack too."

My aunt kept saying, "What's wrong? What's wrong?"

I said, "Nothing's wrong. She's just fainted." I didn't want to alarm my aunt. But I kept my eyes on my watch, and after one minute the pulse returned, and she snapped out of it.

My mother looked up at me, and she said, "You won't believe this, Stanley, but your father just took me by the hand and said he didn't want to die without saying good-by to me."

About 1961, in Portland, Jacob was driving down the street with a friend, Dr. Ben Siegel, Professor of Experimental Pathology. They were on the way to Bonneville to see the hyperbaric chamber.

I told Ben about my father's dream and about the wood rot. This was before DMSO. Ben looked at me; he was sitting on the right side of the car, and I was driving. He said, "Stanley, you're supposed to be a scientist. That's the craziest thing I have ever heard."

As he finished, he looked out the car window, and there on the theater marquee was the title *Follow That Dream*.

Dr. Eduardo Ramírez, the Peruvian scientist who had reported considerable success with DMSO in treating certain mental diseases, wrote to Jacob in June 1971, asking if the FDA ban was still in effect. He told Jacob that the Ministerio of Salud Publica of Chile had approved DMSO for pharmaceutical use in humans, both for topical and intramuscular administration. And he asked if it would be possible to get permission from the FDA to continue his work with DMSO in mental patients, claiming that he thought he had found a way to mask the sulfide odor and at the same time to potentiate the therapeutic action.

Ramírez said the DMSO combinations were being produced and clinical tests sponsored by Laboratorios Recalcine, S.A., in Santiago. Nicolas Weinstein was president of the Chilean concern.

Weinstein had read the article by Jacob et al. in a 1965 issue of the *Journal of the American Medical Association,* and his spirits soared. The editorial in the same issue which cast great doubt on the factuality of the findings failed to quench his enthusiasm. He set about testing DMSO on laboratory animals, domestic animals and humans. By the time the FDA's alarums reached him, Weinstein had confirmed some of the Jacob-Herschler findings and had launched his own broad program.

At his New York hotel on a quiet and rainy Sunday morning in October 1971, Weinstein spread out on the table before me an impressive array of papers and journals, in English and Spanish, extolling the therapeutic effects of DMSO combinations. He had just spent a day or two in Portland with Jacob and now, on his way back to Chile, was full of ideas and zest.

At seventy, the stocky, balding Weinstein was energetic, physically and intellectually. He obviously enjoyed his adventures on the sidelines of science and experimental medicine. He said that he had been trained as a pharmaceutical chemist at the University of Chile, in his native Santiago, had spent fifty years working in the laboratory, and, as president of Laboratorios Recalcine, S.A., he now headed the largest drug house in his country.

Weinstein said his agents ran laboratories in Japan and several countries in Europe. He said that his products outsold those of his competitors on a free and open market. He could—and did—sell DMSO for seventy cents per 100 cc—DMSO which he bought from Canadian sources, which in turn had obtained it from Crown Zellerbach in the United States. He said his great advantage was that he could incorporate drugs produced by others into his combinations, whereas the big international competitors were pretty well restricted to the use of their own drugs. He boasted that he was the first in all the world to offer DMSO as a prescription drug.

Most of the papers on Weinstein's products were of a geriatric bent—on such conditions as atherosclerosis, emphysema and senility. He seemed proudest, however, of advances he claimed had been made against mental retardation. He did not argue that his drugs would transform the village idiot into an Einstein, but he did state that after months of treatment, the three-year-old mentality of a young adult might be advanced to the ten-year-old level. This, he said, is accomplished with a combination of DMSO, and GABA (gamma aminobutyric acid) and another ingredient or two. DMSO, he felt, had not only an additive or multiplying effect on some drugs but detoxified them as well.

He described with glee the harvest of sprains and strains yielded by four hundred Olympic skiers in Portillo soon after he had obtained a supply of DMSO and the miracle of a French woman who recovered from a twisted knee and sprained wrist overnight and who went out and won the gold medal.

He said the castration wound in pigs healed rapidly when DMSO was used; his researchers applied the finding to human tonsillectomy—a spray of DMSO induced rapid healing where one tonsil had been, whereas repair proceeded at the normal rate on the contralateral, untreated, side of the throat.

He described the disbelief of the veterinarians as he cured hoof-and-mouth disease with a spray of mixed DMSO, antibiotics and anti-viral preparations. He outlined his observations of the rapid disappearance of shingles, of asthma, of peritonitis and of burn wounds in humans treated with DMSO combinations. He told how a DMSO combination was sprayed on the throats of hundreds of child victims of a major earthquake six months earlier and how the drug enabled even those with double pneumonia to breathe easily almost at once and to leave the crowded hospitals in about half the time it normally takes.

Weinstein said that intramuscular injections, as well as throat spraying, of DMSO combinations were enabling emphysema patients to increase their activities greatly.

A couple of weeks after our conversation, I received a sizable bundle of confirmatory reprints and their translations authored by researchers in reputable Latin American institutions. The literature suggested indications for use, composition, biochemical mechanisms, dosage and administration methods, side effects and contra-indications. Here are some of the statements and claims of the Chileans—with their uppercase orthography:

MERINEX is composed of 1) several amino acids (GABA, CABOB, acetyl glutamine, L-arginine, aspartic acid) to stimulate nerve cell function and synthesis of proteins, glutathione, and acetylcholine, and to reduce hyperexcitability and spasticity; 2) centrophenoxine, which by regulating oxidation-reduction metabolism of nerves, "improves memory, combats confusion and increases the power of concentration"; and 3) the most important ingredient, dimesuline (DMSO), "acts as a penetrating transporter" and exercises a "tranquilizing, anti-depressive, psychotonic and anti-anxiety action."

The package insert said that MERINEX was indicated for apathy and mental states in the old—depressive neurosis and asthenia in people who are subject to stresses, agitation, irritability, anxiety, suicidal tendencies, disorders of the climacteric, hysterical neurosis, brain and nerve damage, hardened arteries, stroke, apoplexy, and the effects of megavoltage radiation for cancer.

It also claimed usefulness in such symptoms as poor performance in school and bad behavior in infancy and adolescence—mental retardation.

The package stuffer contended that an ampule or capsule every other day wrought almost immediate and long-lasting improvement in many youngsters more than three years old.

In the aged, MERINEX could be injected into muscle or taken orally in capsules for various infirmities.

There were such reports and claims as:

Carlos Nassar, Head of the "Department for Children in Irregular Situations" of the National Health Service of Chile: MERINEX was given to 44 retarded (oligophrenic) children, 21 of whom had forebears with speaking or walking psychomotor difficulties often due to genetic and nutritional deficiencies, brain damage at birth, and other identifiable influences. "Medical pedagogic statistics reveal an alarming increase in school-age mentally retarded."

He quoted the Minister of Education as saying: "In Chile there are some 250,000 homes in which children do not laugh as other children do. They do not talk as other children, nor do they have full educational development such as other children."

Detailed tables indicate these treatment results up to 13 months with every one of the patients tolerating MERINEX "excellently:"
Favorable—60 per cent
doubtful—10 per cent; and
negative—30 per cent.

Successfully treated children showed a significant rise in IQ, accelerated progress in basic efficiency, increase in total intellectual efficiency, progress in reading, writing and mathematics, coordination in movement, better manual ability, improvement in conduct problems, and better psychomotor control with abandonment of unreasonable aggressiveness, irritability and rebelliousness.

Children who received both capsules and injections improved more and faster than those who received MERINEX by one route only.

Still another study of fifty retarded children (that is, their IQ's were under 55) was reported in *Revista Chilena de Pediatría* by Dr. Azael Paz:

> Thirty were given three MERINEX capsules a day orally for about six months; the other 20 were treated similarly but on one day a week they took their MERINEX by intramuscular injection. Scores were by "psycho-pedagogic computation."
>
> After 10 or 15 days of treatment the "process of maturing and learning" began to accelerate in 25 phases of improvement, including the lessening or disappearance of autistic quiet, automatic movements, inertia, passivity, negativism, irrational aggression, rebellion, timidity and withdrawal.
>
> At the same time these traits developed: awakening of the senses, psychomotor drive, activity, acceptance of tasks, interest, initiative, expression, language, control of laughter and anger, group contact, identification and transfer, egocentric attitudes, language enrichment, order, motivation, work, making purchases and eating and dressing alone, attention, spontaneity, reading, writing and drawing.
>
> This group did not include those with serious cerebral damage, as in congenital cerebral paralysis and convulsive epilepsy.

A majority of 48 men and women, ranging in age from 24 to 80 years given MERINEX for diverse neuropsychiatric disorders responded favorably. Drs. Eduardo Brucher and Patricio Torres of the Psychiatrical Hospital in Santiago and Dr. Gustavo Munizaga, Chief Neurologist at the Polyclinic of Neurology and Professor of

Neurology at the University of Chile, described the overall results as excellent in 8.4 per cent, good in 60.4 per cent (they became normal), regular (comparable to results with other therapies or no treatment) in 25 per cent, and no response in 6.2 per cent.

Progress during periods of no treatment was compared with that when they took MERINEX regularly. Improvement was reported in hardening of brain arteries, stroke, hypoxia, spasm or blockage of blood vessels, senile paranoia, dementia and deterioration, alcoholic deterioration, depression (involutive, Parkinsonian, organic, post-typhus), and psychoses following head injuries.

The only objectionable side effect was odor.

DMSO not only exerted tranquilizing, anti-depressive, anti-anxiety and psycholytic effects of its own, but dissolved other constituents of MERINEX and transported them through the blood-brain inside the brain.

Professor Munizaga treated 84 men and women for various psychologic disturbances of old age for an average of about three months with a combination of MERINEX and any one of three other DMSO drugs. About 95 per cent showed favorable responses. The other drugs were Ipran, DIXI-2, and P-92.

Ipran contains DMSO, procaine, hematoporphyrins and two vasodilators—bufenine and tetranitrate of pentaerythritol. Munizaga felt the combination opened blood vessels to and in the brain, and provided for the feeding of undernourished brain cells.

P-29—composed of procaine, hematoporphyrin and Pemoline—served as a metabolic energizer which improved memory and thinking processes.

DIXI-2 is an anti-anxiety drug (due to its diazepam and chlormezanone constituents) and a muscle relaxant and anti-depressive.

The chief neurologist at Hospital San Francisco de Borja, Dr. Jorge Grismali, and Dr. Luis Varel Barrios of Hospital del Salvador reported that 75 of 100 patients with cerebrovascular disease responded favorably (only four showed no benefit at all) to Ipran which was administered orally and by injection. It sped recovery from stroke and relieved stroke-threatening symptoms.

Grismali and Barrios treated another series of 70 men and women at the Hospital del Salvador with MERINEX orally and intramus-

cularly once a day for a week and once every other day for a second
—and, if necessary, third—week.

Their diagnoses were anxiety neuroses, depressive neuroses, hysterical neuroses and intellectual deterioration.

More than one half with various neuroses enjoyed excellent responses to MERINEX: symptoms subsided completely within two weeks, and improvement was long-sustained. Most of the rest had a "good result"; their symptoms came under control within three weeks and remained quiescent for several weeks following therapy.

Those with neuroses lost their anxieties, irritability and aggressiveness; the "chain irritability," which had produced conflicts in the home and at work, was broken; insomnia lessened and suicidal urges subsided in a vast majority, the researchers said.

There were no excellent results of treatment of those with intellectual deterioration, and not quite one half of these patients achieved good results.

With Ipran against mental diseases of old age, Dr. Augustin Tellex, Professor of Psychiatry at the University of Chile, said thirty-eight of forty-five patients benefited.

For the asthmatic syndrome, including bronchiectasis, allergic bronchitis, emphysema, collagenosis and lung fibrosis, Weinstein had compounded two DMSO preparations called Aradix.

White ampules of Aradix containing Aminophylline (or theophylline ethylenediamine) rapidly relaxes bronchial tube muscle and dilates the tube, and water.

The amber ampule, with Chlorpheniramine maleates, contains an anti-histamine to reduce allergy, Dexamethasone phosphate, a potent anti-inflammatory and anti-allergy adrenal corticoid hormone, and water.

The white and amber ampules usually are mixed, drawn into a syringe, and injected very slowly into a muscle.

Drs. Zoltan Bernath, Ernesto Chacon, Norman Bennett and Adriana Rivera tested the preparation on 145 ambulatory and eight bedridden patients at Hospital San Francisco de Borja. The subjects had had symptoms—asthmatic crises, bronchitis and the like—for anywhere from one year to several decades.

In this, as in other Latin American trials described here, the researchers conducted detailed physical and chemical tests periodically over the course of their studies.

ARTROTIN, designed to help arthritis victims, contained DMSO (or dimesuline, as they call it) mixed with a chemical cousin of Butazolidin one called gamma-keto-phenylbutazone, an anti-rheumatism corticoid known as Dexamethasone, and acetyl-glutamine, an important building block in the protein molecule.

Four faculty members at the University of Chile tested ARTROTIN on 122 patients, with scleroderma, arthritis, periarthritis, bursitis, fibrositis, vertebral osteoarthritis or spondilosis, cox-arthrosis, and arthrosis of the knees and hands. They had been treated ineffectively with steroids, analgesics, indomethacin, Butazolidin, vitamin B_1 and hot sulfur and mineral baths.

X-rays and a scoring system showed 80 per cent had a good response, 17 per cent regular, and 3 per cent no benefit.

Despite the fact that all the drugs in this mixture can be severely toxic (DMSO excepted), every patient tolerated treatment well.

Dr. Raul Berrios de la Luz, Assistant Professor of Medicine, was the senior investigator.

Dr. David Sabah Jaime, head of the university's Rheumatology Department at hospitals in Valparaiso, injected ARTROTIN into 40 aging women with chronic rheumatoid arthritis, 3 with disseminated lupus erythematosis, 4 with scleroderma, 2 with psoriatic arthritis and 1 with dermatomyositis. The diseases had resisted treatment with aspirin, corticoid hormones, gold salts and physiotherapy.

68 per cent enjoyed "obvious improvement," 25 per cent moderate improvement, 5 per cent no improvement or progression of the disease, and one patient withdrew following a temporary allergic reaction to the drug . . . a rash that responded to anti-histamines.

All the scleroderma and psoriatic patients received definite benefit.

DMSO seemed to prevent the highly toxic effects of the drug's other constituents.

Weinstein has produced an aerosol which he calls Plus-Par, advertised as anti-bacterial, anti-viral, anti-inflammatory, analgesic and hemostatic. DMSO once again not only lends its own germ-killing properties to this mixture but enables the dissolved drug to penetrate the skin and go to the scene of action in varicose ulcers, pharyngitis, tonsillitis, rhinitis, otitis, stomatitis, herpes of the genitals, lips and back, cervicitis, pyoderma and various surgical wounds.

Cytoglutal, a combination of DMSO, amino acids, and cyclophosphamide, a common cancer drug, was injected into patients with incurable cancers of various sites. This treatment appears less toxic than the conventional drugs and might be a little more effective especially in some leukemias and lymphatic cancers, the investigators contended.

Among Weinstein's other DMSO mixtures were:

Neopon K, for joint conditions;

Neo-Pluripen, for infections; and

Tripsiquim, to prevent arterial and venous thromboses and to reduce their damage.

I asked Jacob how he felt about the possibly extravagant claims of the Latin Americans. He said, "I'd like to be certain."

He went to Santiago to see for himself.

When he went to Chile for ten days in December 1971, Jacob was given a hero's welcome by Weinstein, the numerous physicians using Weinstein's DMSO preparations, by hospital nuns and nurses, priests and patients. During his visit he listened to the doctors and the patients; he lectured to the academicians and students; and he came away with considerable interest in what he had seen and heard.

Jacob returned from Chile a few days before President Nixon signed the Cancer Act of 1971, allotting $1,600,000,000 for cancer research in the United States during the next three years. The signing was done in dramatic fashion, in a ceremony involving fourteen United States Senators and 123 other celebrities drawn from the top names in finance, society, science, industry and, to be sure, politics. It had been a long time since the United States had introduced any important discoveries in cancer treatment, or indeed in any treatment.

Chile spent a total of, roughly, $30 million a year for its entire research and development program. Since it is difficult to support HEW-type, or even FDA-type, bureaucracy with that kind of money, Chile had had to forego the massive propaganda machine, the no-knock police force, the thought surveillance system, and other expensive scientific accouterments of her mighty neighbor to the north.

When Stanley Jacob returned from Chile, he told me, "The articles we have read in the Chilean literature seem fairly solid. Chilean investigators contend that they have made advances against many disparate diseases with DMSO combinations—mental retardation, atherosclerosis, stroke, cardiovascular disease of several types, emphysema, the symptomatology of senility. Their claims should be investigated."

Mrs. Betty Lou King, wife of a Portland Chamber of Commerce executive and a crusader in children's health causes, accompanied Jacob to Chile. The Kings' son, Billy, 14, was called Mongoloid; his features were Asiatic, his tongue large and slightly protruding, his hands shovel-shaped. He had the look of a fetus who had become stranded somewhere along the great journey into this world.

Mrs. King had been profoundly impressed with the progress Billy had been making on a regimen calling for a teaspoonful or so daily of DMSO in his orange juice or tomato juice, while under Jacob's care. After several weeks, his features began to change toward normal; he started to trace letters on paper; and one day he came to his mother and uttered the first sentence he had ever initiated: "I love you."

Her observations in Chile convinced Mrs. King that Billy's improvement—like the miracles which had been reported to her in Chile—was due to DMSO. She began to organize benefits in Portland to support Jacob's controlled study on retardation.

With increasing vehemence over the years, Jacob's friends advised him to stop this nonsense and claim a share of the royalties from his patent rights. He had remained adamant in his refusal on the grounds that the commercial aspect might impair DMSO's chance to win the FDA's acceptance.

Jacob's friends advanced these arguments:

1) He was broke and deeply in debt.

2) He needed funds to fight for DMSO.

3) What would happen to his employees and his able associates, if the economy wave sweeping over research institutions would strike his own projects?

4) What would happen to DMSO, to his patients, to his career in research if he lost control of the fruits of his labor?

The arguments were telling; the last seemed to stagger him. The omission of his name from bibliographies in papers on DMSO and even from the forty references cited by Syntex in announcing the advent of Domoso, its veterinary DMSO, reminded him that scientific credit can be short-lived.

A series of events brought the patent royalties matter to a head late in 1970. The medical school faced a financial crisis; the state Board of Education was reported ready to distribute medicare and other funds, not only to the medical school, but more generally. It was becoming clear that royalties from DMSO might be handled in a similar manner—despite Jacob's desire to see them used by the medical school and, especially, by the Department of Surgery.

The first royalties from Syntex's veterinary Domoso soon would be due. Friends warned Jacob that while the state would look with favor now on the idea of splitting royalties with Jacob, this generosity well might subside when real money was at hand. As his chief, Dr. William Krippaehne, put it: one third of nothing is nothing and easily given away; one third of something is different.

Herschler, too, faced a crisis. Crown had given him a check for $500, presumably "fair compensation" for one of his patents—one for a DMSO anti-perspirant preparation. (Jacob said this patent had no utility—"it substituted one odor [DMSO] for another [body, underarm, etc.]"—and would have none until DMSO was rendered less smelly.) Herschler was not cashing the check, lest his acceptance of it be considered as approval of the arrangement. Meanwhile, without a laboratory, or a secretary, or duties, he was passing time in the Crown library. He was given more $500 checks for more patents; and these too remained uncashed.

Herschler saw Jacob's lawyer, Norm Kobin, and inquired about the possibility of diverting some of the royalties into a non-profit organization to be called Search, Incorporated. Under such a set-up, Herschler would like to explore other plant chemicals, and Jacob would test DMSO on human diseases which were incurable, rare and so medically unprofitable that drug houses would not invest in their research.

At the urging of his associates in surgery and others at the medical school and at the invitation of Freeman Holmer, Vice-Chancellor of the Oregon State System of Higher Education, Jacob on June 17, 1971, finally asked for 30 per cent of the Board's royalties for himself and 70 per cent for the medical school.

The state, acting through its Board of Higher Education on behalf of the University of Oregon Medical School, readily conceded in a flurry of "hereinafter's" and "whereases" and "now, therefore," that Jacob, as co-inventor (the other co-inventor was Herschler), would receive 30 per cent of the state's net patent income.

The patent rights estimates were running as high as nine and ten figures. With about 100 different patents applied for or granted in various countries, Jacob said that Herschler and he would share, as partners, all money either man derived from DMSO, and if it were enough, both would spend the rest of their lives in research of potential benefit to mankind.

I asked Jacob if he had applied for a patent on DMSO's ability to restore hair. He said he had not. This could be one of the most lucrative of the DMSO patents.

"There is no doubt now that DMSO stimulates hair growth," he said. "It has done so—very slowly to be sure—in almost every person we've tried it on.

"We've been applying DMSO for the last eight months to save a gangrenous hand," he said. "The patient still has dry gangrene, but pictures of the two hands show the one receiving the DMSO has significantly more and longer hair growth than the other hand.

"At meetings, the veterinarians report the hair grows on animal limbs treated with DMSO better than on the untreated limbs."

With the passage of time, the flow of literature on DMSO was increasing steadily. Because perhaps 90 per cent of the research was done abroad, it came to Jacob largely through the Library of Congress. It dealt with a very broad spectrum of pathology.

I have abstracted some of the papers as follows:

RHINOSCLEROMA

Rhinoscleroma, caused by the bacillus Klebsiella, starts usually as a non-tender little lump in the nose and spreads as a stony mass to involve the breathing tubes and sinuses. Surgery, even effective, can be as mutilating as the disease.

DMSO dissolved the polysaccharide capsule coating the bacilli and permitted any of several antibiotics to destroy them; the combinations enhanced patients' normal resistance to the bacteria between 128 and 4,096-fold.

In one series, all 25 patients were cured. Diseased mucous tissues began falling away during the second week of treatment, and the solutions were dabbed or sprayed onto the wound. A combination of DMSO and prednisolone was used to prevent scar tissue from forming in the respiratory tract.

Long-continued monitoring of the patients showed no acute ill effects of treatment on the blood, urinary tract, respiratory system, eyes and ears. [R. A. Barilyak et al., Lvov Medical Institute, *Polish Literature*, 1968]

TEETH

Researchers at the University of Bern conducted controlled studies of pulpitis treatments for ten years. Pulpitis is inflammation of the central part of teeth, the part containing the nerve and blood vessels.

DMSO alone improved 75 per cent of the cases; and DMSO plus oxyphenylbutazone (a drug for gout) or chloramphenicol improved 85 per cent, as compared with 50 per cent of those on placebos. [H. Triadan, *Medicine and Hygiene*, 826 bis/May 22, 1968]

EARDRUM

DMSO was applied in the ear in 20 cases of eardrum surgical repair, in which the patient's own tissues were grafted to form a new membrane. The operations were successful in 85 per cent.

Outstanding features were the absence of post-operative perforation, sloughing of the graft, dermatitis, scar formation, adhesions and fungus infections. No internal ear damage was found. [S. K. Vishwakarma, Aligarh Muslim Univ., India; *Plast. Reconstruction Surg.* 42(1) (1968): 15–17]

HEART PROTECTION

A total of 240 rats were given isoproterenol subcutaneously on two consecutive days. This caused portions of the heart muscle to die and decay, as sometimes occurs following a heart attack.

Surviving animals were divided into three groups: 1) one was given no treatment; 2) one was given 0.5 ml of 90 per cent DMSO subcutaneously daily; and 3) the other group was given distilled water instead of DMSO. The animals were killed and autopsied at various times.

The water-treated and DMSO-treated animals showed hearts less damaged than those of the untreated, so far as necrosis was concerned. Moreover, the DMSO-treated showed not only less damage than the untreated, but the injury was of a different, milder, sort; and in them there was no evidence of heart muscle rupture or aneurysm.

The research was done in 1965 at Walter Reed Army Medical Center, but no journal would publish it at that time because of the FDA's attacks and ban on DMSO. [Arthur S. Leon (Newark Beth Israel Hospital) et al., American Association of Pathologists and Bacteriologists meeting, May 1969]

LOCAL AND GENERAL EFFECTS

A total of 125 tests were made on 69 patients, most of them with a broad assortment of rheumatic conditions and a few of them with conditions resulting from trauma. DMSO 84 per cent was brushed generously on either 1) the affected area, or 2) a distant site. Results were graded on the basis of none, moderate or good pain relief.

Therapeutic success was recorded for 65 per cent of applications at the site of complaints and 60 to 61.6 per cent for distant applications. A rubbing agent, used as a control, achieved 11.1 per cent success when applied at a distant site.

The results showed DMSO has a generalized systemic effect. [H. von der Hardt et al., Robert Koch Hospital near Hannover, *Med. Welt*, March 11, 1969]

DNA VIRUS INFECTIONS

DMSO with IdU (5-iododeoxyuridine) cleared up skin lesions caused by DNA viruses and it prevented recurrence.

The treatment worked well, and in some cases spectacularly, on herpes simplex and zoster, chicken pox, and vaccinia. Among the

37 cases, every one showed healing in about one third the normal time.

Fresh cases healed rapidly and often completely. Older simplex cases took longer to heal and tended to recur; however, if the recurrence was treated promptly, healing was very rapid and there was no tendency toward further recurrence.

The only "sequelae" reported was post-healing pain for three and seven weeks and six months in three of the eleven zoster patients. (Many shingles patients suffer pain for years after the clearing of their lesions.) [R. C. Turnbull et al., Otago Univ., Dunedin, *New Zeal. Med. Journal*, 70, 317; 11/69]

PERIODONTAL DISEASE

A total of 32 men and women 18 to 45 years old with periodontal disease were treated with DMSO.

In 13, the disease appeared restricted to bleeding and swollen superficial layers of the gums. In the other 19, oozing and painful pockets of infection extended deep into the gums, sometimes involving bone and loosening teeth.

Following diagnostic x-rays, teeth cleaning and repair, microscopic examination of gum samples, blood and fluid tests to identify germs and other sources of disease, the patients were treated with compresses containing 30 per cent DMSO applied to the outside of the gums for ten minutes during each of seven to ten visits on alternate days. Twenty non-diseased people, as controls, were similarly treated.

"Remarkable improvement"—total elimination of pain, decreased bleeding, and gum adherence to teeth—occurred in all patients with superficial disease. All patients with deep infections reported less inflammation and disappearance of painful symptoms, but in none did very loose teeth firm up. Controls experienced no untoward reactions. [Prof. Dr. J. Krzywicki, Head of the Clinic of Behavioral Stomatology Medical Academy, Warsaw, Poland, *Czas Stomat* XXII:LL (1969): 1007–10]

PAIN

DMSO 84 per cent was applied, in a double-blind study of 69

patients with injury or rheumatic pains, to 1) near to or 2) far from the site of pain. Results: 65 per cent of the "near-to" and 60 per cent of the "far-from" pain site patients reported good results. Only 11 per cent of the (non-DMSO) control subjects reported good results. [H. von der Hardt et al., Med. Klin. Robert Koch Krankenh., Land Hannover, *Med. Welt* 20(11) (1969)]

ARTHRITIS

Croton oil was injected into the knees of rabbits, inducing arthritis. DMSO then was injected into the arthritic knee. The sooner the injection, the more favorable the results. [R. Suckert, Univ. of Vienna, *Wien Klin. Wschr.* 81(9) (1969)]

SKIN AND NERVE CONDUCTIVITY

DMSO 40 per cent in salt (9 per cent) distilled water decreased skin electrical resistance by about 100 per cent, thereby increasing nerve conductivity. [S. J. Turco and A. T. Canada, Temple Univ., *Amer. Jnl. Hosp. Pharm.* February 1969]

CATTLE INFECTIONS

Cutaneous staphylococcic infections of cattle were treated successfully with daily applications of flumethasone and penicillin dissolved in 90 per cent DMSO. [F. Vitali, Univ. of Parma, *Clin. Vet.* 92(12) (1969)]

VETERINARY MEDICINE

Of 171 domestic animals with varied diseases seen in veterinary practice, 146 were cured and 17 improved. [K. H. Schaeffler, Staat Tierarztpr. Kühlungsborn, Kreis Bad Doberan; *M.H. Veterinaermed.*, August 15, 1969]

SKIN

DMSO plus 5-iododeoxyuridine, applied to the affected skin areas, gave good to excellent results in 20 patients with cold sore virus infections, shingle virus in 11, two with eczema and one each with warts and chicken pox. [R. C. Turnbull, Otago Univ. Med. School, Dunedin, *New Zeal. Med. Journal*, 70(450) (1969)]

TEETH

Experiments with radioactive DMS^{35}O show that the solvent penetrates dentin, except for sclerotic tissue. The observation suggests the possibility that DMSO might prove useful in root canal treatment and in therapy for pulp gangrene where, as a vehicle for other drugs, it might exercise a bactericidal influence. [Franziska Fruh-von Arx, Interlaken, *Schweiz Zahnheilk*, November 1969]

PAIN

DMSO, alone and in combination with hydrocortisone, novocain or edan, was applied to the skin overlying painful areas in 76 patients with diseases of rheumatoid origin, inflammation of nerve roots or spinal disc problems. For experimental patients, 85 per cent DMSO was used; in control patients, 1 per cent DMSO.

As compared with control patients, those treated with 85 per cent DMSO began showing improvement as early as one hour after treatment, with the greatest improvement after three hours. In some cases pain disappeared completely. Within one week of treatment improvement was recorded for 5 of the 8 rheumatoid patients, 17 of 20 cases of inflammation of nerve roots, and 8 of 10 people with disc pains.

All DMSO treatments were superior to conventional therapy. DMSO was most effective when given with hydrocortisone, novocain or edan. [Jacek Glazewski, Tarnow, *Polish Literature*]

NERVE REGENERATION

DMSO, with 1–3 per cent phenol combined with hyaluronidase, the enzyme known as the "spreading factor," was injected around the sciatic nerves of rats, who were observed clinically for six weeks, and then sacrificed and examined histologically.

Weakness and paralysis were proportional to the concentrations of phenol or DMSO injected. Myelin and axon destruction also depended on the concentrations of DMSO and phenol. But "the findings confirm the relatively few reports indicating that peripheral nerve will regenerate" and that, following nerve damage by 100 per cent DMSO, "nerve fiber repair occurs fairly rapidly." [Leslie W. Knott et al., Stanford Univ., *Neurology*, Vol. 19, October 1969]

RADIATION PROTECTION

Dabbing DMSO on the skin did not protect against the effects of x-rays. Neither did DMSO plus mercaptoethylamine or epinephrine. [R. F. Hagemann et al., Univ. of Iowa, *J. Invest. Derm.* 52(3) (1969)]

RADIATION PROTECTION

Acute radiation burns were inflicted on the shaved skins of rabbits, who had been paired for experimental purposes—one served as offering an area for DMSO treatment, the other presenting burns treated with a prednisolone-DMSO mixture. A third group was treated with trihydroxylethylrutoside solution, or THR.

Close studies of the affected epidermis (with stains) showed a distinct reduction in inflammation of areas treated with DMSO/ THR and a rapid healing and regrowth of damaged tissues, as compared with DMSO alone or DMSO plus prednisolone. THR is a bioflavinoid, vitamin P. [K. H. Kärcher et al., Univ. of Heidelberg, *Germ. Med.*, 1969]

PEA PRODUCTION

Sprayed on the leaves of "Dark Skin Perfection" peas, DMSO (5 per cent) increased the yield of peas 11.3 to 25 per cent. Cycocel increased the pea yield 14.6 per cent and 17.4 per cent. And DMSO plus Cycocel showed an additive effect of the two growth constituents. [A. R. Maurer et al., Canada Dept. of Agriculture, Agassiz, B C; *Hort. Science*, Vol. 4, Winter 1969]

PLASTIC SURGERY

Skin grafts, even with tissue removed from one side and transplanted to another site on the same body, often fail. Evidently, proteolytic enzymes become active and destroy the graft moorings. Dressings moistened with 30 per cent DMSO solution enabled grafts to take and survive in badly burned patients and victims of elephantiasis. [M. F. Kamaev, Lvov Medical Institute; *Klin Khir* (Kiev), 5 (1969): 65–67]

EAR TROUBLE

A simple procedure was tested successfully in 69 patients, 37 girls and 32 boys, with otitis media, or inflammation of the middle ear, and 17 with inflammation of the maxillary sinus.

A 30–50 per cent solution of DMSO was poured into the cleaned ear and put under slight pressure. The solution, sometimes containing an antibiotic, usually penetrated to the eustachian tube, bathed it, and passed out into the nasopharynx. In suppurative otitis media, there was rapid cessation of suppuration, or pus discharge, return of hearing and normalization of the blood.

In purulent inflammation of the antrums of Highmore, 30–50 per cent DMSO was given by puncture. Cures were achieved in a majority of cases within 4–8 days; and the results of treatment usually were long-lasting. [Ia. M. Golod, Soviet Union, *Zhurnal Ushnykh, Nosovykh i Gorlovykh Boleznei*, 4 (1969): 65–66]

ANTIBIOTICS

The antibiotic substances sodium fusidate and fusidic acid, with DMSO penetrate the skin at a rate seen with glucocorticoids. [C. F. H. Vickers, Liverpool Univ., *Brit. J. Derm.* 81 (12) (1969)]

CATARACT PREVENTION

Irradiated mice developed cataracts. If they were treated with DMSO—given topically to the eyes—8 minutes before 1,000 R to the head, lens opacification was not complete. While the lens was protected by DMSO, the cornea may have been made more radiosensitive. [R. F. Hagemann, Allegheny Gen. Hosp., Pittsburgh, *Radiology* 92 (1) (1969)]

FUNGUS INFECTION

A patient with an infection of the foot by M apiospermum which was unresponsive to antifungal agents rejected amputation. He was treated through an indwelling catheter to the infected area two hours a day for 16 days with amphotericin B (and later Fenticlor) dissolved in 60 per cent DMSO. The patient improved and was discharged; no serious side effects were noted.

Four months later, the patient was treated for a recurrence, which was found due to a complicating bacterial infection. The leg was amputated; and examination and tests showed no fungi present. [C. Edward Buckley III, et al., Duke Univ. Med. Center, *Arch. Intern. Med.*, December 1969]

PARONYCHIAE

Dr. Hans Weitgasser in the district hospital in Gras, Austria, treated 38 cases of chronic paronychiae (inflammation around nails) with a combination of DMSO and TA, triamcinolone acetonide, a cortisone-type hormone. He achieved excellent results in 21, good in 12; and he controlled the disease in all but 2.

Even in 20 cases complicated by infection with candida, yeast-like organisms, good or excellent results were obtained in 15.

In many cases, the TA was incorporated in VOLON-A tincture— a 2 per cent alcohol solution with 0.05 per cent benzalconium chloride, a wetting agent with antiseptic properties, 2 per cent salicylic acid, and TA—which was dabbed on the affected area followed by 90 per cent DMSO.

Paronychiae often follow hangnail trauma in which micrococci, fungi or detergents penetrate the skin, and they are most common among pastry cooks, dishwashers and housewives. Weitgasser found many of his patients were diabetic or had pre-diabetic conditions.

Conventional treatment—hot compresses, the surgical draining of purulent pockets, the application of antibiotics and cortisone-type hormones, and removal of nails which necessary quite often is not very effective against long-standing cases. [*Zschr. Haut Geschl.-Krkh.*, Vol. 44, 1 (1969): 27–30]

TUBERCULOSIS

Thirty-two patients with destructive pulmonary tuberculosis complicated with TB of the bronchi and non-specific endobronchitis were treated with 10 per cent and 25 per cent DMSO solutions of streptomycin and penicillin, by inhalation and endobronchial infusion.

Most of the patients improved, and 14 ceased excreting TB mycobacteria. DMSO may be a useful auxiliary treatment in antibiotic-resistant disease. [V. I. Lyubinets and M. V. Kruk, Lvov, *Postunnula* 10, 11 (1969)]

BULL PENIS INFECTION

Trichomonas foetus is a common and costly infectious agent among cattle. It is very difficult to cure in infected bulls. Until now, it has been necessary to massage the extruded bull penis and foreskin for 20–30 minutes with an antibiotic ointment while instilling a solution into the urethra. A single surviving organism can lead to recurrence of the infection, and the procedure must be repeated in 10–14 days.

Test-tube experiments showed that DMSO alone killed trichomonads; and so did acriflavine. When DMSO and acriflavine were combined the two drugs exercised a multiplying effect on each other in their trichomonicidal potency.

Twenty-three infected bulls were tranquilized, and each was treated by: 1) instilling a liquid containing 0.5 per cent acriflavine and 50 ml DMSO into the urethra, while at the same time 2) wetting the exposed penile mucosa with an acriflavine-DMSO ointment. The procedure took 3–5 minutes.

All bulls five years old and under were cured. Only about 40 per cent of the bulls older than six years could be cured by this method. [M. A. Hidalgo et al., Syntex Research, Palo Alto, Calif., and Mexico, D.F., *Veterinary Record*, August 8, 1970]

SKIN CANCER AND PRE-CANCER

DMSO 70 per cent and then 5-FU ointment were applied to ten patients with senile keratoses—the type of skin liver spots which some consider pre-cancerous—basal cell cancer in one, and several areas covered by an inherited skin-scaling condition known as xeroderma.

While the combination caused many of the lesions to clear up after several days of treatment, the elapsed time and follow-up have been insufficient for accurate evaluation of the therapy. [A. Garcia-Perez, Salamanca Medical Faculty, *Dermatologica* (Basel) 140 (Supl. 1) (1970)]

TEETH AND GUMS

DMSO 30 per cent was applied to inflamed areas around bad teeth. Inflammation cleared up in all 32 patients so treated. [H. Rewesska, Klin. Stomat Zacho, Warsaw, *Czas Stomat* 22 (11) (November 1969)]

CHICKEN VIRUS

Weak DMSO (0.5 to 1.5 per cent) had contrary effects on two related but different chicken viruses—herpesviruses which cause Marek's disease. The experiments were carried out on chicken kidney cells grown in glass dishes and infected with either Type I PPA virus or Type II PPA.

DMSO, when added in extremely small amounts, to the culture greatly inhibited PPA I's ability to infect the chick kidney cells. On the contrary, DMSO in the same amount increased the infectivity of PPA II. [T. Mikami and R. A. Bankowski, Univ. of Calif., Davis, *Am. J. of Vet. Res.*, 1970]

PLASTIC SURGERY

Skin flaps were cut surgically on the backs of rats. Several agents were tested for their protective effect against necrosis of the flap. DMSO offered some small protection. Hyperbaric treatment—putting the animals in an oxygen-filled tank under two or three times normal pressure twice a day for two days—was a little more effective.

The experiments ended after two days. [G. Arturson and N. N.

Khanna, Burn Center and Department of Plastic Surgery, Univ. Hospital, Uppsala, *Scand. J. Plas. Surg.* 4:8–10 (1970)]

PARKINSON'S DISEASE

Controlled experiments in rats showed that L-dopa, the drug used with considerable success against Parkinson's disease, can be dissolved in DMSO and be transported into the brain where it is altered into dopamine, the active form of the drug. Another relative of L-dopa, called 5-HTP, also can be dissolved by DMSO and carried into the brain where it becomes active as dopamine. Dopamine can not cross the blood-brain barrier; the only way it can enter the brain and do its good work is in the form of L-dopa or HTP—and then let an enzyme in the brain (a decarboxylase) change it into active dopamine.

Efforts have succeeded to a degree in knocking out carboxylase on the blood side of the barrier. This is done with a chemical monkeywrench called DCI (decarboxylase inhibitor) which permits L-dopa and HTP to roam freely through the blood without fear of being changed to dopamine until it crosses the blood-brain barrier.

Using fluorescent stains, scientists have injected 1) L-dopa, 2) DMSO to transport it into the brain, 3) DCI (in this case called nialamide) designed to prevent blood carboxylase from changing L-dopa into dopamine; and they have been able to trace the L-dopa into brain capillaries and the nervous tissue where it became dopamine and turned off the brain functions which bring on the trembling and other symptoms of Parkinsonism.

This work so far has been done in rats. But because, in this particular phase of body chemistry, rats have behaved a good deal like humans, there may be hope for improved treatment of Parkinsonism. [J. C. de la Torre, Univ. of Chicago, *Experientia* 26, 1117 (1970), Birkhauser Verlag, Basel]

SYSTEMIC LUPUS ERYTHEMATOSUS

DMSO plus fluocinolone were given to a woman in whom chloroquine and high doses of prednisone had failed to control systemic lupus erythematosus. Eye symptoms developed. The hormone was withdrawn, and the eye symptoms subsided. On DMSO alone, the patient achieved a complete remission which, so far, has lasted three years. [M. Brandsma et al., Los Angeles; *Angiology* 21 (3) (1970)]

INTERSTITIAL CYSTITIS

DMSO 50 per cent (but not 100 per cent) proved safe when instilled in large volumes into animal bladders every two weeks for as long as six months.

This simple and inexpensive treatment has effectively controlled symptoms for as long as five years in about two thirds of patients with interstitial cystitis. [B. H. Stewart et al., Cleveland Clinic Foundation, in press, 1970]

TRAUMA

DMSO 80 per cent was applied to injured knees, upper legs, rib cages, shoulders and other areas four times a day in 36 patients. Side effects included skin reddening after three applications, skin peeling after six, a dermatitis after six—all of which disappeared soon after withdrawal of DMSO. Healing generally was rapid. [M. B. Dubinsk and A. A. Skager, Riga Medical Institute, 1970]

HERPES ZOSTER

DMSO containing a dye was applied to a pig "for the skin of this animal is most like that of a man," and the combination passed through the whole thickness of skin. Human tests then were undertaken.

Idoxuridine 5 per cent in DMSO greatly reduced the pain and sped healing in several groups of patients with herpes zoster, or shingles. Idoxuridine 40 per cent in DMSO continuously applied for four days gave much better results, especially in patients older than 60 years; pain, which normally lasts more than one month, was gone in less than three days, on an average, healing was greatly accelerated, and recurrences were rare. DMSO-idoxuridine treatment appears to prevent post-herpetic neuralgia. DMSO alone and idoxuridine alone were without great benefit. [B. E. Juel-Jensen, Oxford Univ. Clinical Med. School, Annals N. Y. Academy of

Sciences 1731, Article I-74, 1970, Second Conference on Antiviral Substances]

HERPES VIRUSES

An ointment containing DMSO and deoxyuridine was applied to 46 patients with various herpes infections. The same ointment with the hormone, prednisolone, added was given to another group of 57 herpetic patients. Both preparations produced good results in an average of 3.8 days. Local irritation occurred in four patients in each group. [Th. Nasemann and Falco O. Braun, Univ. of Munich, *Ther. Gegenw.* 109 (2) (1970)]

ANTI-INFLAMMATION

DMSO applied to the skin improved experimental contact dermatitis and allergic eczema induced in guinea pigs with dinitrochlorbenzol. In rats and guinea pigs, DMSO reduced skin inflammation and skin death due to allergic reactions. [Iren B. Kovacs, Otto Korvin Hospital and United Pharmaceutical Works, Budapest, Hungary, 1970]

"SMART PILLS"

PMH (magnesium pemoline) has been claimed by others to have improved learning in rats and in humans. Pemoline dissolved in 100 per cent DMSO greatly increased rat learning ability over levels achieved with pemoline alone.

Radioactive (carbon-14) PMH dissolved in water or dissolved in DMSO was injected into the bellies of rats. The DMSO/PMH was from 50 to 100 per cent more successful in crossing the barrier from blood into brain than was the water solution. [John J. Brink and Donald G. Stein, Clark Univ., *Science*, Vol. 158]

SHINGLES

Shingles, a painful and sometimes extremely serious infection of nerve roots, is caused by herpes zoster, a relative of other herpes viruses which cause simple cold sores, chicken pox, a blinding eye disease, and infections of male and female genitalia which sometimes are associated with cancer of those organs, especially of the uterine cervix.

Shingles brings blisters of pinhead size to pea size, which follow the course of the infected nerve. Nerve (neuralgic) pain can be intense and long-lasting during the acute stage; and, especially in older people, a torturing postherpetic neuralgia may persist for months or years after the last blister has burst and dried up.

Oxford scientists wet strips of gauze with 40 per cent idoxyuridine and 100 per cent DMSO and kept them continuously over the sores of 22 zoster patients. The strips were rewet daily. In a median of two days—and nine days at the latest—the pain disappeared, and healing was accelerated.

The results were similar in uncontrolled and two double-blind clinical studies. [*British Medical Journal*, 4 (1970): 776–80]

ANTI-VIRUS

Many anti-cancer preparations proved too toxic in the doses needed to kill cancer. Some, however, proved useful otherwise. One of the drugs—IdU or 5-iododeoxyuridine—proved highly effective against herpes, the viruses which cause shingles and cold sores and which bring complications which sometimes can cause blindness, insanity and death. IdU had drawbacks: It did not penetrate the skin well; it was toxic; and the infection often recurred. When DMSO was mixed with IdU, the complex penetrated the skin rapidly, was effective in small, mild doses, and often appeared to knock out the virus for good. Similar benefits were achieved with the DMSO/IdU combination in other virus infections, including varicella, vaccinatum, atypical warts, and eczema herpeticum. [R. C. Turnbull et al., Otago Univ. Med. School, Dunedin, New Zealand]

MECHANISM OF DMSO ACTIVITY

The groin of a cow was painted with DMSO; the cow was slaughtered and the tissues viewed under the microscope.

Mast, or fat, cells had erupted, releasing granules of histamine, which makes capillaries more permeable and sets off an allergic-like inflammation, and 2) heparin, the anti-coagulant. Apparently,

DMSO dissolves and diffuses heparin, histamine and some other blood and cell contents and together with its heat-generating effect, softens and dissipates scar tissue, and activates the defensive lymphatic cells known as the reticuloendothelial system, or RES. This may be the means by which DMSO erases scars, enhances immunity and speeds regeneration. [Dr. Bertalan Simonkay, *Hungarian Veterinary Journal*, 26 (6) (June 1971)]

ADRENAL HORMONES

DMSO plus adrenalin injected into the jugular vein of very young chicks concentrated 34.8 per cent more adrenalin in the brain than did injections of adrenalin alone. Similar results were achieved with DMSO plus noradrenalin—in this case, DMSO increased the brain concentration of noradrenalin 38.8 per cent. [Joseph P. Hanig et al., U. S. Food and Drug Administration; *J. Pharm. Pharmac.*, 23 (1971): 386–87]

HERPES SIMPLEX

Two potent antirheumatic drugs, mefenamic acid and indomethacin, proved to be effective treatments for herpes virus when applied with DMSO over the affected areas.

The preparations were put up in small bottles and given—along with instructions on their use—to staff members of the Institute of Immunology and Experimental Therapy and patients attending the dermatology clinic. The patients themselves applied a few drops of the drugs every two or three hours for one day or longer when herpes lesions appeared, most often on the lips, but also on the face, nose, mouth and genitals.

Incomplete box scores on 64 patients show that either DMSO-indomethacin or DMSO-mefenamic acid, when applied early, clear up most eruptions in 2 to 4 days, in contrast to the 10 to 14 days for untreated cases to clear up. In some, but not all, recurrences became much less frequent. Both mixtures showed anti-viral and anti-inflammatory activity in patients with no more than 2 per cent strength of indomethacin or mefenamic acid.

The mixtures in even lower strengths—0.12 per cent mefenamic acid and 0.18 per cent indomethacin in 5 per cent DMSO—demonstrated virus inactivation in vitro. DMSO at 5–20 per cent concentrations may have shown a protective influence on viruses (against freezing), but at room temperature DMSO alone in these concentrations did not suppress or protect the virus. DMSO 40 per cent and stronger, however, almost completely inactivated the virus. [Anna D. Inglot and Aleksandra Woyton, Institute of Immunology and Experimental Therapy, Polish Academy of Sciences, Wroclaw, *Archivum Immunologiae et Therapiae Experimentalis* 19,535 (1971)]

RINGWORM

The antibiotic, griseofulvin, will not cure ringworm, and DMSO alone will not cure ringworm.

But a paste of griseofulvin tablets in DMSO cleared it up completely in 5–10 days in cats. [H. B. Levine et al., Naval Biomedical Research Laboratory, Univ. of Calif. School of Public Health, *Sabouraudia* 9 (1971): 43–49]

FUNGUS INFECTIONS OF NAILS

Griseofulvin in DMSO cleared up severe fungus infections of toenail—and in some cases fingernail—areas, and new nails grew after 6 to 12 weeks of treatment. [Tadeusz Checinski, Dept. of Dermatology, Bieganski Hospital, Lodz, Poland, Meeting of Lodz Division of Polish M.A., September 1971]

INTERFERON PRODUCTION

When viruses attack tissues, cells produce an anti-viral substance called interferon. The interferon slows or completely arrests the virus invasion.

White mice were injected with two kinds of viruses, and their production of interferon was measured. Vienna scientists discovered that if DMSO was injected 10 minutes after the mice were infected with the viruses, the animals produced anywhere from two to 16 times as much interferon as they normally would following infection. [M. Kunze et al., Zbl. Bakt., *I. Abt. Orig.* 216 (1971): 527–31]

RADIATION

DMSO protected cancer patients against the dermatitis—including erosion, blistering, itching and pain—caused by high energy rays. It also appeared to enhance sensitivity to the radiation and accelerate regrowth of normal tissues.

When one side of an irradiated area was given DMSO protection and the other side not, the protected side showed fewer ill effects. DMSO therapy was withdrawn in only one of 22 patients because of an eruption which was thought possibly due to DMSO. The fact that DMSO-treated areas showed skin reddening and exfoliation earlier (and more mildly) than untreated areas indicates that DMSO may have sensitized these tissues to x-rays; but DMSO also sped recovery. The skin darkening effect of x-rays was greater in the DMSO-treated patients.

The patients had cancers of the uterine cervix (12), breast and upper jaw (4) and breast and cervix (6). [Goro Irie et al., Hokkaido Univ., Sapporo, Japan]

HORMONE ABSORPTION

The adrenal cortical hormone, hydrocortisone, was dissolved in DMSO, and measurements were made of the time it took to be absorbed through the skin; and clockings showed that the higher the concentration of DMSO (in a range of 12.5 to 100 per cent) the faster the hormone moved. The tissue content of hormone built up gradually during when given at two-hour intervals for 16 hours. Pig skin was used in these experiments. [D. G. Perrier and J. N. Hlynka, Univ. of Alberta, Edmonton, *Canadian Journal of Pharmaceutical Sciences*, Vol. 5, No. 4 (1970)]

MICROCIRCULATION

DMSO 60 per cent was brushed onto the inner forearm of patients, and, with the aid of such instruments as a thermistoral thermometer, a digital plethysmograph (to record pulse volume), a capillary microsocpe and other fine instruments, many pre-DMSO and post-DMSO measurements were made.

DMSO raised the skin temperature 1.2° Celsius in 10 minutes, due in part to brushing; pulse volume rose 10 per cent; capillary vein diameter increased 12 per cent; microcirculation increased around scars.

DMSO, in increasing local microcirculation, caused no suggestion of undesirable side effects. [Pal Daroczy and Eva Ladanyi, Medical Univ. of Debrecen, *Review of Dermatology and Venereology*, Vol. 46 (1970)]

FRIEND LEUKEMIA VIRUS

Cells containing a leukemia virus (Friend) were grown in glass dishes. When 2 per cent DMSO was added to the culture medium, the cells developed differently than they did when DMSO was not present. For one thing, they looked more like the normal cells which eventually give rise to good healthy red blood cells—maturation or differentiation, the normal "growing up" process is called. The DMSO-treated cells had their protein-producing structures (ribosomes) altered from those found in cells capable of inducing leukemia in mice; and evidence of hemoglobin synthesis tended to confirm opinions that DMSO might have a sort of "normalizing" effect on the cells.

The DMSO-treated cells contained numerous "budding" viruses. It is possible that the DMSO, by a chain of biochemical events still unknown, interrupted the cell's virus-manufacturing or virus-releasing processes. [Toru Sato, Charlotte Friend and Etienne de Harven, *Cancer Research* 31 (October, 1971): 1402–17]

C-TYPE VIRUS

Cells removed from a human muscle cancer were grown in a glass dish. The cells did not produce viruses.

When an anti-virus drug, 5-iododeoxyuridine (IdU), was added to the culture medium, a few virus particles appeared inside the cells.

When DMSO also was added to the medium, the production of virus particles inside the cells increased ten-fold. (DMSO alone—without prior IdU—had no effect, however.)

The viruses were found budding from the endoplasmic reticulum

—large masses of protein-producing ribosomes. Whether the viruses mature, leave the cells, and infect other cells is not known.

A similar phenomenon was induced with IdU and DMSO in another cancer—a tumor of the glandular tissue of a human lung. In this case, those peculiar, changeable particles called mycoplasma, or PPLO, were also present. "As contaminants," the scientists said.

Questions remaining to be answered are:

1) Do the viruses or PPLO cause cancer?

2) Does the appearance of viruses represent a step toward cell maturation and non-malignancy?

3) Do the PPLO particles inhibit the virus? Are they contaminants?

Other scientists earlier had shown that IdU alone will clear up some herpes simplex (cold sore) virus infections of the eyes—a very serious condition in many instances. And a combination of IdU and DMSO will do a much better job. [Sarah E. Stewart, et al., Georgetown Univ., and Theresa Ben, National Cancer Institute, *Science*, December 16, 1971]

VETERINARY MEDICINE

Perhaps the most widespread trials of DMSO in veterinary medicine up to the time of this report was on 171 domestic animals—cattle, pigs, horses and dogs—with a variety of diseases. Of the 171 treated with DMSO, 146 were cured and 17 others improved. Only 8 animals appeared uninfluenced by the treatment.

Treatment was simple—most often the topical application of 75 per cent DMSO to large animals and 50 per cent to small ones. It was safe—little or no serious toxicity was observed. And in some cases, it was spectacular—animals which could not be helped by other means and with a poor prognosis occasionally responded rapidly to DMSO alone or in combination with other drugs.

In cattle: Postpartum mastitis often disappeared with two rubbings after milking. Acute panaritium, or foot rot, with its pain and lameness healed in 3–8 days. DMSO proved more effective than diuretics in some cases of edema.

In pigs: Sows with mastitis became normal sometimes within hours of the first udder massage with DMSO, and they allowed their piglets to suckle. The anti-inflammatory and bacteriostatic properties of DMSO were impressive in preventing ill effects of boar castration.

In horses: Horses with lumbago showed an almost normal gait often just a few hours after rubbing with DMSO; muscles regained their softness and elasticity. Three days of treatment made the animals useful again, as a rule. Lameness due to several causes yielded to DMSO.

In dogs: Painful disc injuries healed rapidly. Eight of nine dogs with painful paresis of a hind leg were cured with DMSO—in six of them in less than five days. Generous paintings with DMSO 2–3 times daily cleared up eczema in less than a week.

The scientists have drawn up the appended table indicating the variety of diseases encountered and the results of treatment. [K. H. Schaeffler, Staat Tierarztpr., Kühlungsborn, Kreis Bad Doberan, *Pharmakologie,* 1969]

Animal species	Diagnosis	Number of cases	Duration	Better	Cured	No influence	Remark
Cattle	Non-purulent acute mastitis	18	3-5 days	17	1	—	+ antibiotics
	purulent mastitis	5	1 week	5	—	2	
	acute crown-toe or mid-toe panaritium	11	1 week	11	—	—	pour-on cast
	shoulder lameness	7	1-2 weeks	7	—	—	after jumping
	gonitis	4	1 week	3	1	—	
	traumatic carpitis	2	1-2 weeks	1	1	—	
	purulent tarsitis	1	3 weeks	1	—	—	
	tendovaginitis	3	1 week	2	1	—	
	purulent pododermatitis	7	1-2 weeks	7	—	—	pour-on cast
	hematoma	5	1-2 weeks	4	1	—	
	birth edema	3	1-2 weeks	3	—	—	
	herpes tonsurans joint distortions	9	3-5 days	9	—	—	effective but could not be evaluated
		77		69	6	2	
Pig	acute puerp. mastitis	13	3-5 days	10	3	—	
	chronic mastitis	3	1-2 weeks	2	1	—	
	avoidance of wound swelling after castration	10	3-5 days	8	2	—	slight swelling
	lameness after distortion	5	3-5 days	2	2	1	
		31		22	8	1	

Animal	Diagnosis	n	Duration				Remarks
Horse	lumbago	5	3–5 days	5	—		moderate
	tendovaginitis, acute	5	3–5 days	5	—		
	tendovaginitis, chronic	2	3 weeks	—	2		
	chronic peritarsitis	2	3 weeks	2	—		
	shoulder lameness	2	1–2 weeks	2	—		+ spavin-iron pour-on cast
	bursitis carpalis	1	1 week	1	—		
	podotrochlitis	1	3 weeks	1	—		
		18		16	2		
Dog	discopathy	8	3 ds.–5 wks.	7	1		
	intervertebrate enchondrosis	1	6 weeks	1	—		with X-ray control
	eczema madidans	7	3–8 days	7	—		
	mycoses	2	1 week	2	—		
	idiopathic lameness	5	1–4 weeks	4		1	with X-ray control
	gonitis ossificans	2	2 weeks	2	—		
	perica pitis ossificans	1	1 week	1	—		
	muscle rupture	1	3 weeks	1	—		
	purulent conjunctivitis	4	2–3 weeks	4	—		10% solution
	cataract	2	4 weeks	—		2	30% solution
	primary glaucoma	1	3 days	1	—		30% solution
	external purulent otitis	5	3–5 days	4		1	
	hematoma	5	1–3 weeks	2		1	
	stand-up ear surgery with Perlon implantation	1	1 week	1	—		for wound healing
	mastitis puerperalis	2	3 days	2	—		
		45		39	1	5	
	summary	171		146	17	8	

Part Five

At fifty-six, Jack Brandis had just about everything—a charming wife, a loving family, a good mind, handsome mien, a luxurious home high on a mountain overlooking Portland, a new Lincoln Continental among his cars, a fine athletic record at Oregon State, membership in the best clubs, a low handicap, an army of friends and admirers, many million dollars and terminal cancer of the prostate, with a prognosis of maybe a week at the outside.

He also had courage; he wanted very much to live.

It was his cancer and courage which caused Brandis's family to seek Jacob's services. And for some time it looked as though a camel might go through the eye of a needle before this rich man could enter Jacob's clientele. There were many reasons for barring Brandis: he was bedridden; any number of physicians could usher the dying man into the hereafter; Jacob had no special competence for such a case and no desire to undertake at this time a special study of hopeless cancer patients; and, above all, there was the problem of time—Jacob's waking hours already were overcommitted.

The trouble is that Jacob finds it virtually impossible to say no to anyone; and when Brandis's emissaries finally did penetrate his defenses, Jacob said reluctantly, "Well, I'll look at him; but I don't believe there's a thing I can do for him." Brandis's personal physician was not encouraging. He pointed out that the cancer had progressed relentlessly since its diagnosis seven years earlier. The patient had been put on the female hormone estrogen—one of several endocrine procedures devised by the great Nobel laureate Dr. Charles B. Huggins of Chicago, which greatly improved the lot of patients with hormone-dependent cancers. With Brandis, there had been prostatic resection but no castration; and colonies of cancer now were riddling his bones. The femur in his right upper leg had snapped; and there was extreme pain where x-rays had shown other bone erosions—in the chest, back, pelvis, both legs. He was paralyzed from the waist down. His frame, once large and muscular, was emaciated and waterlogged.

Brandis lived at home; his large, luxuriously furnished bedroom had been rigged with the most modern hospital devices.

Dr. Jacob, on his first visit, looked down on the dying man, then in a partial coma, and he resolved to be firm—he would decline as gracefully as possible to enter this case. Then Brandis opened his eyes, and, as he tried to extend his large, bony hand, he grinned.

"Thanks," Brandis said. "You saved me a lot of trouble."

"How?" Jacob asked.

"By coming here today," Brandis said. "Otherwise I would have bought the medical school and ordered you to come."

At the end of his visit, Jacob said he would review the literature on DMSO in cancer. "If I feel then that DMSO will help at all, we'll give it a try," he said.

Beyond the unconfirmed claims of the Chilean clinicians, there is considerable evidence that DMSO, alone or in combination with other agents, might prove helpful against some cancers. The evidence is highly circumstantial but impelling. It is possible that no other compound, in its basic biochemical behavior, shows as much specificity against cancer as does DMSO. This is not to say that in DMSO the cure for all cancers is at hand. An enormous amount of study is needed to determine DMSO's proper place in medicine's weaponry against the scores of malignant diseases categorized as cancer.

DMSO's strongest hints of anti-cancer activity have come from studies in leukemia—cancer of the blood and blood-forming bone marrow and lymphatic tissues.

Dr. Robert Schrek and associates at the Veterans Administration Hospital in Hines, Illinois, once made movies of normal and leukemic cells under attack by various anti-cancer drugs. The cells were stained with eosin and placed under a phase contrast microscope. A cell "census" was taken before and after onslaught by each agent added to the culture.

Schrek found that x-rays destroyed cells of chronic leukemia and, more readily, those of acute leukemia. The trouble was, even in very small doses of radiation, normal useful lymphocytes were sometimes killed; and in other cases, both the normal and leukemic cells proved resistant to x-rays. Cortisone-type hormones also killed leukemic cells much more readily than normal cells, especially in chronic lymphocytic leukemia.

A temperature of 109.4° F for two hours proved more toxic for leukemic than normal cells, but a lower temperature (107.6° F) had equal lethal effect on both types. The findings raised again the century-old suggestion that high fever may be nature's way of suppressing cancers.

The most selective treatment of all, however, was DMSO. It was active in the low concentrations attained in the bloodstream. Two per cent DMSO, which had no effect on normal cells after two days, killed 90 per cent of the leukemic cells in a single day. Even patients in remission presented cells highly sensitive to DMSO. The Schrek group felt that the DMSO effect might be specific enough to indicate whether or not a lymphocyte donor had leukemia.

The husband-and-wife team Drs. David and Martha Berliner of the University of Utah, with Dr. Thomas F. Dougherty, Professor of Anatomy, dissolved a cortisone-type hormone in DMSO and added the solution to cultured fibroblasts, young, fiber-spinning cells. The cells quickly shriveled up. A similar solution did the same to leukemic cells in culture—and then in leukemic mice.

At about this time, a little girl in Salt Lake City had come to the end of the line. She had had a good response to x-rays—then to cortisone—then to methotrexate. And then she stopped responding to any of these or other treatments given her. She was bleeding, her mouth was ugly with sores, she was in pain and obviously dying. The scientists applied the DMSO-steroid combination, and it did no immediate good. But they treated her again—and again—and again. And in a few days, they had both objective and subjective evidence that she was improving. Within a few weeks the girl was back in school and at play. She was well for almost a year before she relapsed. The DMSO-steroid combination gave her a second long remission. Then when leukemia again recurred, the treatment was tried once more; but it had lost its magic. The girl died. At this time DMSO was banned by the FDA, and the Utah group stopped using it even on cultured fibroblasts.

For many years scattered scientists—mostly women—have been finding TB-type or leprosy-type dwarf bacteria associated with cancer—including human cancer. Some believe that the organisms cause cancer. The peculiar particles are called variously Progenitor cryptocides (a member of Actinomycetales) L-forms, Lister forms, mycobacteria, PPLO (pleuropneumonia-like organisms), protoplasts, spheroplasts, mesosomes, pluripotential or pleomorphic organisms. They assume more forms during their development than science has thought up names for them; at various stages they may resemble viruses, bacteria, molds, films, filaments, fungi, motile rods, discs, dots, balls, eggs, biscuits, blobs and other structures. Their diet—the content of the culture—influences their size and shape. They are kin to the germs in BCG, the vaccine against tuberculosis and cancer.

While the mycobacteriologists do not agree with one another in every particular, their work is generally mutually confirmatory. They include Dr. Irene Corey Diller of the Institute for Cancer

Research, Philadelphia; Dr. Florence B. Seibert, formerly of the University of Pennsylvania and now of the Mount Park Hospital Foundation, Inc., St. Petersburg, Florida; Dr. Virginia Wuerthele-Caspe Livingston of La Jolla, California; and Dr. Eleanor Alexander-Jackson of New York.

Not only have they isolated the organisms from numerous urine, blood and tumor specimens of cancerous animals and humans, but they have infected animals with them and produced cancers, immunized animals to a limited degree and discovered some substances which seem to discourage cancer development.

Seibert, in a wide-ranging search for natural and synthetic compounds with anti-cancer activity, tested DMSO against her dwarf bacteria and the cancers they caused. When she examined blood specimens, fifty-nine cancer patients yielded the suspect organisms, which were then grown in culture dishes. She found the organisms also in 80 per cent of the normals who had visited cancer patients; presumably they had been infected but resisted the agents.

Seibert and her associates (Frances K. Farrelly and Catherine C. Shepard) discovered that lysozyme, one of the body's common and potent defenses against infection, had very little influence over her organisms; in fact, when it showed any activity at all, it stimulated as well as suppressed their growth. Ethambutol, a powerful poison used against tuberculosis resistant to other treatments, also had limited effect on the organisms when used alone, but it did seem to potentiate the high doses of lysozyme.

When the Seibert group added 12.5 per cent DMSO to cultures of organisms isolated from sixteen of eighteen cancer patients' tumors and blood, their growth was completely inhibited for thirty days; in control tubes there was marked growth. Seibert's discovery that the hardy, drug-defying dwarfs can be both weakened and killed by innocuous doses of DMSO encourages speculation not only that DMSO may find a place among anti-cancer drugs but also that it may lead to an anti-cancer vaccine.

After her paper was published, Seibert wrote Congressman

Wendell Wyatt of Oregon: "The possibilities for benefit from DMSO to cancer victims should certainly be explored with great energy, especially when one balances any hypothetical harm it may cause with the toxicity of many of the drugs now used against cancer."

Dr. Leo Stjernvall, a University of Helsinki pathologist, and his associate Dr. K. Setala, a veteran cancer investigator, have reported that anti-cancer drugs will penetrate deep into normal cells and benign tumor cells and halt their growth. Cancer cells, however, build a protective "cytoplasmic barrier" which prevents the poisons from seeping inside the cells and killing them or arresting their growth.

Stjernvall dissolved the anti-cancer drug vinblastine sulfate in DMSO and dabbed it on cancers that he had induced with chemicals applied to the mouse skin. The fibrous cytoplasmic barriers melted away, and other structures changed so that the cancer cells took on the appearance of benignly overgrown but otherwise normal cells. Other common anti-cancer drugs became equally effective when dissolved in DMSO.

The experiments showed that DMSO-transported drugs can alter the malignant cell toward normal. The experiments tended to confirm the early observations of Dr. Edmund Klein of Roswell Park Memorial Institute in Buffalo that the anti-cancer drug 5-FU, in DMSO will clear up 90 per cent of the (basal cell) skin cancers and pre-malignant keratoses in patients.

Dr. Titus C. Evans of the University of Iowa, one of the early users of isotopes to measure metabolic rates, and Dr. Ronald F. Hagemann, now of Pittsburgh, Pennsylvania, showed that DNA, or gene substance, is manufactured by mouse cancer (S-180) cells at a reduced rate in the presence of DMSO; the stronger the DMSO the slower the cancer growth.

Purdue investigators Drs. Chung-yi Chang and Edward Simon discovered that DMSO depresses the growth of HeLa, tumor cells which have grown by the hundredweight in test tubes all over the world since the original tumor was removed a generation ago from a very sick Baltimore black woman. They also found that DMSO suppressed disease-causing viruses.

Dr. J. Ernest Ayre, a New York cytologist, had contended that intrauterine devices bring about cervical cellular changes resembling those seen in precancerous and cancerous states. He said that DMSO makes these and other early cancerous lesions disappear.

Dr. Charlotte Friend, the noted virologist, and her associates at New York's Mount Sinai School of Medicine and the Sloan-Kettering Institute for Cancer Research have transformed leukemic cells back to normal, useful, hemoglobin-manufacturing cells, with a very weak concentration (2 per cent) of DMSO added to the medium in which the cells were growing. The scientists had cultured blood-making cells which produce a virus strong enough to induce leukemia in some mice but weak enough to immunize others against the disease. Because others had shown that DMSO enhances the infectivity of the RNA core of viruses (polio and mengo) and transforms the ubiquitous cancer-causing polyoma virus, DMSO was used with the objective of superinfecting the leukemic cells with Friend virus. Again, DMSO did the opposite of what was expected—mice injected with DMSO-treated leukemic cells outlived those receiving untreated cells by a very wide margin, and the tumors grew much slower with DMSO added to the inoculum.

In April 1973, Drs. Etienne and Jennie Lasfargues of the Institute for Medical Research, Camden, N.J., reported that while DMSO increased the number of virus-infected mouse breast cancer cells sixfold for a while, by the end of three months DMSO had completely rid the cultures of infected cancer cells. Following this, the surviving cells had developed thick membranes, possibly a protective measure.

A few years ago William V. Siegel, then a fourth-year dental student and now a D.M.D., and Gerald Shklar, D.D.S., Professor of Oral Pathology at Tufts School of Dental Medicine, set out to speed up the induction of cancer in hamsters with one of the most potent carcinogens known to man—DMBA, or 9, 10-dimethyl-1, 2-benzanthracene. The way to accelerate the action of DMBA, they reasoned, was to dissolve it in DMSO and to paint the hamster's cheek pouch with the solution. Or, they thought, if they painted the pouch with DMSO and then applied the DMBA, they might produce cancer instantly. The hormone triamcinolone, was added to increase the size and invasiveness of induced cancers.

The investigators were amazed. Instead of speeding up the cancer induction, DMSO slowed it down or suppressed it completely.

Chewing betel nut is generally suspected as the cause of the great many mouth cancers among Far Eastern populations. There has been no certainty about this, however, since no one has been able to induce cancers in laboratory animals with betel nut or with any of the many materials in it, including cured tobacco and other organic and inorganic chemicals.

Dr. Kailash Suri and his associates at Boston University felt that DMSO might dissolve any cancer-causing chemical in betel nut preparations and induce in the cheek pouch of hamsters cancers similar to the tumors found where humans hold a betel nut quid. They painted various test solutions on the hamster cheek pouches three times a week for twenty-one weeks. They found that DMSO (which by itself has never caused cancer in any animal) induced neither cancer nor leukoplakia, the precancerous pearly lesions. DMSO plus tobacco yielded leukoplakia but no cancers in 8 of 12 animals; DMSO plus betel nut resulted in 19 cases of leukoplakia and 8 of cancer in 21 hamsters; and DMSO plus tobacco and betel nut gave 18 cases of leukoplakia and 16 of cancer in 21 animals.

If the results of these laboratory experiments were extrapolated to man—something few scientists would attempt—they would indicate that while DMSO itself is perfectly innocent, it might dissolve and activate cancer-causing chemicals and combinations of

334

them. And, because many of the agents used to treat cancers are themselves carcinogenic, it is not unreasonable to suppose that DMSO might enhance the anti-cancer effect of these drugs—as shown by Stjernvall, Morris Green and others in mouse studies.

A group of scientists at the University of Maryland discovered that DMSO dissolves the pigments which protect aflatoxin-producing fungi from destruction by ordinary ultraviolet light. (Aflatoxin in food is a potent carcinogen.) When the investigators, headed by Dr. G. A. Bean, added a touch of DMSO to the culture medium, the green pigment of the spore-making conidia drained away; and when the fungi then were exposed for only thirty seconds to ultraviolet light, every last one of them stopped reproducing and died out. The fungi which were not exposed to DMSO, and which consequently retained their pigment, were much harder to kill; 30 per cent survived and they repopulated the culture with pigmented offspring.

These experiments, in this case with strains of *Aspergillus flavus*, suggest that DMSO might make other organisms radiation-sensitive—including those which produce cancer in turkeys, the mycobacteria described by Dr. Seibert, and fungi infecting plants, animals and humans.

The Maryland group found that a low dose of DMSO in culture (5,000 parts per million) made the fungi increase production of aflatoxin; beyond that, however, the higher the concentration of DMSO the less the aflatoxin, until at 50,000 ppm the fungi produced 1 per cent or less of the normal amount of aflatoxin.

Back in 1967, FDA Commissioner Goddard, told the fifty or sixty journalists covering the American Cancer Society's Seminar for Science Writers of the numerous steps involved in making a cancer cure available to the American public. As an estimate, five to ten years would elapse, during which time between 1.5 and 4 million Americans would die of the disease.

"Protecting the patient—even the terminal patient—still comes first," the commissioner said. "The [Food, Drug and Cosmetic]

Act requires FDA to stop clinical studies to protect patients, if we believe this is necessary. In the area of experimental cancer drugs we will continue to take firm and appropriate action to protect all patients. Where clinical testing is done in secret, we will extend ourselves to the utmost to determine the facts and take prompt action."

He described as essential to the patients' protection the mass of reports, the reams of IND data . . . all the information that has been generated by the investigational drug program . . . including the clinical records of all patients treated with the drug . . . all the information from the laboratories and clinics, from the scientific literature here and abroad, and from independent investigators.

"Safety is not enough," he added. "The drugs must demonstrate a benefit-to-risk ratio weighted in favor of the patient. Effectiveness in drugs has a special meaning for the cancer patients. It protects them from worthless nostrums.

"An NDA [New Drug Application] must contain detailed information on the methods, facilities, and controls to be employed by the drug manufacturer. This assures the patient getting the proper product formulated with the proper composition under suitable conditions of manufacturing, packaged in an appropriate container, and properly labeled."

Jack Brandis couldn't afford the time the FDA demanded.

Jacob studied the clinical reports on Brandis, and he found no comfort in them. The radiologist reviewing the x-rays had said he had never seen a human body so shot through with metastases. Bones were badly depleted of marrow. Brandis not only had no appetite, but it was difficult to find a vein whole enough to permit IV feeding.

Jacob consulted friends who specialized in cancer, and especially prostatic cancer; and they proposed approaches which already had been tried and found futile. He had been impressed by the Chileans' contention that DMSO tended to detoxify standard drugs—this was supposed to permit higher, more effective and safer doses. He decided that if he were given time, he would test this possibility.

First of all, Jacob put Brandis on two ounces of DMSO in fruit juice daily; from experience, he expected this to reduce pain in the thoracic spine. Brandis was still surviving after one week of this oral administration; there was a measurable level of DMSO in his blood; he said his pain had been relieved somewhat.

At the end of the second week, Brandis was drowsy less often, and he commented that he was thinking more clearly. He was outliving the expectancy doctors had conceded him, but it didn't mean much. He was very sick.

As time passed, however, he was able to take ever-more-intense chemotherapy—Oncovin, methotrexate, thioTEPA, 5-FU, Cytoxan, a long-lasting estrogen, and, of course, DMSO. All drugs except DMSO were given intramuscularly; it was still hard to find an accommodating vein. Eventually, Brandis was also given orally 90 million units of a German enzyme complex with vitamins A and E, highly purified and concentrated in emulsion form, which were reported to be yielding very satisfactory results in Europe.

During the early weeks, Jacob drove up to the Brandis home as often as three times a day to make tests and plan the treatment. Then, with objective signs of improvement—the return of appetite, normal eating, diminished edema, the recalcification of bone, and the dispensing with enemas and catheters as normal bowel and urine function returned—Jacob's visits became more occasional. The day Brandis noticed function (sweating) return to his paralyzed legs, he decided to buy a turbo-prop which would enable him to monitor activities in his far-flung timber empire. And that was the day he told Jacob, "With my other cars and the plane, I have no use for my seventy-two Lincoln Continental —it's all yours." Jacob declined, saying he had never accepted a fee for his services and he wasn't about to start now.

People didn't say no to Jack Brandis. On one of the (numerous) occasions when Jacob's second-hand Rambler wouldn't start and he returned to the Brandis home to call the AAA for help, Brandis implored him: "My life depends on the ability of that rattletrap of yours to get you up here. Your car's failure to start could mean my death." The uncomfortable Jacob accepted an Oldsmobile and promptly started seeking a charity to donate it to when, for one reason or the other, Brandis would cease being his patient.

Jacob's therapy had extended Brandis's stay on earth about six months at this time. But the patient was the only one who thought he'd become well again.

While much of the population was sleeping off Saturday night celebrations, Dale Moon and Dr. Latham Flanagan, Jr., rose from their beds at Timberline Lodge, dressed, ate hastily, packed and at a quarter past three on the morning of Sunday, December 27, 1971, set off in a light but steady drizzle that soon turned to sleet and snow. God willing and the weather permitting, they would struggle to the 12,245-foot top of Mount Hood, see what was to be seen, descend and be back at the Lodge before 4:30 P.M., when the sun was to set.

The weather was a party to no such program. Stinging snow was blown by eighty-mile-an-hour winds when the men reached the summit ten hours after they had set out. From their panoramic perch atop the world, they could see a distance of about fifteen feet. It took five days to fight their way back to the lodge. They were frostbitten, dreadfully hungry and too weak even to shiver. They were taken at once to the medical school.

Krippaehne, Chief of Surgery, thawed Flanagan and Moon out. Jacob called the FDA in Washington and talked to an FDA physician.

"Of course you may apply the DMSO, if in your clinical judgment it is indicated in this emergency," said the official.

"How about the IND application?" Jacob asked.

"Make it out at your convenience, and send it in."

Jacob was overjoyed by the ease with which the matter was resolved.

Flanagan and Mr. Moon did beautifully. Their frostbite, moderately severe, cleared up in a spectacular way.

"The most memorable part of all was discovering a real physician in the FDA," Jacob said. He declined to identify the doctor for fear of getting him into trouble with his superiors.

If the FDA relaxed its rigid rules on any other occasion to provide for DMSO treatment, the evidence is hard to find. Nevertheless, piteous appeals were directed by a multitude of patients to the FDA, directly or through congressmen from all parts of the United States. A small sampling included:

I'm quite sure my husband is alive today because of this drug. In March of 1963 he became so bad with gout, he could not raise a hand. He was flat on the hospital bed for 5 months. Every joint in his body was twice its size. He was on strong morphine which could not keep the pain down. Our doctor held little hope for his life. We heard of DMSO and got him to Portland. On DMSO he started improving and at the time the FDA cut off all activity with the drug he was on his feet again and completely without pain. Oh, please God, if Dr. Goddard could only suffer for just one month as my husband suffered for years.

My brother has arthritis of the spine. He is in pain and bedridden more than half the time. When he is treated with DMSO, he is able to lead a normal, active life. If you could live with us for even a few hours, you would understand. The mental anguish of my mother, my brother's wife, and other family members is not a subject I can describe on paper. Just ONE application of this cheap, *safe* DMSO changed my brother from a grimacing patient into an active pain-free man in exactly 30 *MINUTES!* This could come under the heading of "too bad—sad case" *IF* my brother were an isolated case. Multiply him and my family thousands of times, *THEN* think what the FDA's Divine Right of Kings law is doing to thousands and thousands of helpless patients and their families.

My son-in-law suffers from scleroderma. His children weep; my daughter weeps and prays; I weep, and pray, and write letters. Something *must* be done for him and thousands of agonizing citizens. Think how much of our strained budget could be saved by healing these good people and returning them to the land of the living—earning money, paying taxes, being useful citizens once more.

I had arthritis for four years gradually getting worse until I got to the place where I was in such agony day and night I was almost at my wit's end. I had shots in my shoulder joints, x-ray treatments, physical therapy, even a shoulder irrigation, all to no avail. Two doctors—an orthopedic surgeon and an internist—finally said there was nothing more they could do for me except prescribe pills— Emperin codeine which in my case gave only short relief. I heard of Dr. Jacob and went to visit him. I knew DMSO was a brand new drug on an experimental basis, but I would have been willing to try it if it killed me. Almost from the first I began to get relief. Now I am on my feet well and active. I do all my own work and gardening. I have never in my life wished ill of anyone, but experiencing the caliber of this agency (the FDA), I wish every last one of them would suddenly have an attack of acute arthritis so painful you could hear them yell from there to here and have to beg for the only drug ever discovered that could give them real help.

Both as a scientific worker and as a patient with a disease for which no effective recognized therapy exists, I have become increasingly concerned about the manner in which new drug applications are being handled. DMSO has been virtually regulated out of use by the most stringent restrictions on the sale, shipment and use, and utterly prohibitive paper work requirements for investigative use by clinicians. This is in spite of the fact that no authenticated cases of injury to humans have been documented. It would appear that FDA's cavalier treatment of DMSO (and the patients who desperately need it) stems from (a) the publicity it received as a wonder drug in the public press during 1964–65 and (b) the utter impossibility of writing a use authorization at once sufficiently broad to cover the demonstrated indications and dosages and sufficiently narrow to satisfy FDA's concept of its role as the sole arbiter of drug usage in the United States.

In obtaining DMSO for me, you have handed my life back to me, and I am, together with my entire family, grateful. I'm still running a fever, but it's coming under control. My living would not have been possible without your helping hand.

(Pumpian of the FDA, when asked about DMSO, wrote to one senator: "No drug in recent times moved more rapidly from novelty to nostrum than DMSO." When another senator requested amplification, Pumpian assured him, "By our reference to DMSO as a 'nostrum' we were not referring . . . to a 'quack remedy,' which is one of the definitions of the word 'nostrum,' but rather we used the word in the sense of one of its other definitions—that of a 'questionable remedy.' ")

Hope did not die easily or soon with some patients. One woman wrote Jacob in 1971:

My husband has been an experimental user of DMSO for four or five years, having been introduced to it by a Los Angeles doctor. When we went to him about six years ago, we were at the depths of despair. My husband already had had disc surgery ten years earlier—which was completely un-successful—and has been suffering from severe back pain ever since. He shuttled back and forth from doctor to doctor—from physical therapist, to psychiatrist, from hypnotherapy to self-hypnosis, constantly existing on drugs, with nothing giving him permanent freedom from pain.

At the doctor's suggestion, he became an experimental patient for DMSO, and it became his staff of life. He used it for four or five years with complete success, his pain mysteriously or miraculously gone within 15 or 20 minutes from the time of application. (He had many times been so crippled and bent and in pain that he lay

342

on the floor, unable to get up until I applied the miracle liquid to his body. He incidentally never had any side effects.)

And then one day we were told that DMSO was taken off of research and would be available no more.

Dr. Jacob, we are again at the depths of despair. My husband is again crippled and in constant pain. He is about to quit his job.

He would like to become one of your experimental subjects for DMSO. Desperately—

As 1972 drew to a close, the mounting literature made it seem certain that DMSO, sooner or later, would have to be made available to the public. The FDA, facing the inevitable need to explain why it had withheld DMSO, had wished off the embarrassment on the National Academy of Sciences/National Research Council, Science's Hall of Fame, which had served with honor and dignity in resolving some of the nation's most pressing problems since the time of Lincoln.

The NAS/NRC accepted in 1966 an FDA assignment to review evidence of the efficacy of 3,000 drugs which had been introduced between 1938 and 1962. It did so reluctantly, because its decisions and recommendations might be expected to conform with the often impractical parameters set by the FDA. The National Academy may have gone along with the FDA's cry for help only because if it did not undertake this dirty job, another agency might be created to do so. When I discussed the DMSO matter with one NAS officer, he was frank in saying, with considerable heat, "We have been asked to wash the FDA's dirty linen, and we have agreed."

The NAS/NRC review of DMSO literature, conducted by a panel of scientists, would take four months to plan and somewhere between eighteen and twenty-four months to carry out.

In view of the enormity of the evidence, the cost would be a multiple of the money required for a similar study of the average drug.

I asked about this at a press conference for Dr. Philip Handler, the scholarly and sensitive president of the NAS, in April 1972. My question was leading: "As one who has read all the available DMSO literature, I feel that a fast reader could do the job in two weeks and a slow scanner, like myself, in three. Instead of holding up research with the drug for about two years while a panel studies the material—which seems to contain no scientific evidence of toxicity to any humans—why not set three fast readers to work on it and free the drug within two weeks, if no reason is found to continue the ban?" I suggested that the FDA be required to set before the reviewers any solid evidence of toxicity, while Jacob and DMSO proponents be invited to produce all the literature, favorable as well as unfavorable. (Inasmuch as the FDA had not recognized merit in DMSO, it could be presumed to be unaware of the more than 1,200 publications on its benefits.)

Handler responded without hesitation to the Philadelphia lawyer-type question: "I did research on DMSO for Squibb, before DMSO was withdrawn. Consequently, I have taken no part in the matter before the Academy. The answer to your question is 'No comment.'" He was a conscientious man avoiding suspicion of a "conflict of interest."

As DMSO's star rose, the FDA's destiny seemed to decline. Washington watchers found that the agency became involved in ever more ridiculous situations. Like the aspirin crisis.

With those who knew the FDA best saying aspirin would never have made it past that bureau's erratic regulations, it may have been inevitable that aspirin and the FDA should meet on the field of honor. They did. Aspirin lost.

Scientists had noted that a single aspirin prevented the clumping of those sticky little blood cells called platelets, an early event in the clotting process which seals wounds.

Dr. Harvey Weiss, in Roosevelt Hospital, New York, injected clot-inducing chemicals into the carotid arteries of dogs and found that a little aspirin prevented the blocking of these vessels to the head. Dr. Richard Gorlin and other Harvard doctors gave aspirin to patients who had artificial heart valves and greatly reduced disastrous clotting tendencies, although there may have been a theoretical risk of "rebound" clotting.

Until 1971, aspirin had never been used to prevent strokes and heart attacks, so it became necessary to obtain the FDA's blessing, in the form of an IND, to conduct animal and human studies to determine whether aspirin would live up to its initial promise, of reducing the dreadful death rates from these diseases. Dr. William S. Fields of the University of Texas, who had found evidence that "little strokes" are due not so much to narrowed arteries as to small clots, applied for an IND to see whether he could avert cerebral disaster in stroke-prone patients. The Harvard group also wanted to test the effectiveness of aspirin in a series of patients suffering from an insufficiency of blood to the heart muscle, and, because of its urgency, they had started this potentially lifesaving work.

Months dragged on, and when Fields finally cried out in frustration at the American Heart Association meeting in November 1971, the FDA still had not gotten around to his appeal for an IND.

The FDA had taken care of the Massachusetts studies, however; it stopped them because the scientists had not obtained an IND to give the patients aspirin.

Consistent only in being inconsistent, the FDA, a little later, ignored appeals that aspirin/antacid combinations be reformulated. Dr. J. Donald Ostrow of the University of Pennsylvania told the Senate Select Committee on Small Business that he had seen the drugs induce hemorrhage in eighteen ulcer patients in eighteen months; and he suggested, according to the New York *Times*, that Alka-Seltzer advertisers should be made to put on television "a guy vomiting blood and a gastroscope being put

346

down, and where it all comes from." The FDA settled for a warning on labels and in advertising.

At this time, I was asked to pay $11.59 for a small container of pHisoHex—$1.59 for the skin cleanser and $10.00 for the doctor's prescription for the hexachlorophene-containing liquid.

The FDA was broad-minded in permitting some carcinogens, teratogens and just plain filth in food. After a good deal of pressure from consumers and the press, the Federal Register, on March 29, 1972, carried a list of Commissioner Edwards' dirt "defect levels . . . below which the defect is unavoidable under current technology and present no health hazard." The FDA permitted such filth as two rodent hairs or fifty insect fragments in 100 grams (about three ounces) of peanut butter, ten fruit fly eggs or two larvae in 100 grams of tomato juice, and ten rodent pellet fragments in 100-gram samples of cornmeal. The FDA had kept these tolerances secret for more than sixty years.

The food industry, like the drug industry, stood in need of expert guidance, and it too hired FDA employees as they picked up their government pensions and retired. Billy Goodrich had become president of Shortening and Edible Oils, an association whose fifteen members were regulated by the FDA. Billy's old FDA job at the same time was filled by Peter Hutt, a friend and an attorney, who had resigned the job that Billy now took over. In effect, they had swapped jobs.

United Press International quoted Benjamin Rosenthal, a Democratic Congressman from New York, as commenting: "It's an outrage! It's shameful, disgraceful, pitiful! At a time when government integrity is being challenged, high level people are engaging in this musical chairs game where they may favor a special interest." Both Goodrich and Hutt explained that they would avoid cases they had handled in their previous jobs. Hutt declined to name the consumer product manufacturers and associations he had represented on the grounds that it would be unethical to identify them, UPI said.

I had talked with Goodrich a year or so before he moved over into the industrial job. In response to my questions, he told me —a bit sharply—that he could not and did not moonlight, nor was he a consultant, nor had he ever accepted a fee for helping introduce a drug. He said he had no earned income other than the paycheck FDA had paid him for thirty-two years, except for stipends for teaching classes at George Washington and New York Universities. He denied that the FDA's failure to permit DMSO treatment for cats, dogs and humans showed a prejudice in favor of horses. He promised to send me evidence when I begged for proof of "even a single instance of human toxicity." All he sent—and that after some nagging on my part—was an old copy of the Fountain Committee proceedings and still another copy of the non-informative "white paper."

Former Commissioner Ley, whom I contacted at the same time, believed as Goodrich did. He was still hazy about his facts but he felt that DMSO had not been proved safe and efficacious.

I asked Ley how he was getting along, and he answered, "Well, so far—knock on wood—I'm managing to pay my bills doing some consulting work . . . with an industry group—in the new drug area."

When I told Ley that I couldn't think of a single significant drug that hadn't first been introduced abroad in the last ten years, he said, "You're right on that." The most recent important American-conceived drug he recalled offhand was a tranquilizer introduced ten or fifteen years earlier. "The number of native drug inventions have been relatively few recently," he said.

Paul de Haen, the authority on drugs, told me early in 1972 that he too could not remember a really top-notch drug invented and introduced in the United States since the polio vaccines sixteen years earlier.

The data in de Haen's *New Products Parade* had shown that the number of American new drugs had declined steadily over the last decade, while countries like France, West Germany, Italy and Japan were competing for the prestige the United States had abdicated. This was at a time when American consumption of drugs was establishing a new record every year. Evidently the citizenry would take any drug available. Especially tranquilizers.

During the 1960's under toughening FDA restrictions, the number of single new drugs and duplicate single drugs and combinations had dropped precipitously. *New Products Parade* registered a small and brief rise during 1970, a period in which several hundred old drugs had been found ineffective by the National Research Council and taken off the market.

Two of the sixteen single "new" drugs introduced in the United States in 1970 were significant: levodopa (L-dopa) for Parkinson's disease and lithium carbonate for mental disease. L-dopa experimental treatments of humans were first reported in Montreal and in Vienna as long ago as 1961; American scientists improved the dosages in 1967; and finally, in 1970, the FDA permitted Parkinson's disease patients to enjoy this blessing. Lithium salts were used for assorted diseases since the middle of the nineteenth century; and their value in mental disease was reported by an Australian, Dr. John J. F. Cade, back in 1949. It took thirty years to persuade the FDA to permit the use of this drug, which deters some psychotics from suicide.

C. Joseph Stetler, President of the Pharmaceutical Manufacturers Association, said that of eighty-four products developed by American pharmaceutical houses between 1962 and 1972, a total of forty-seven of them were sold in European drugstores before they reached American shelves. Stetler presented figures which indicated that the American lag behind Europe in the introduction of new drugs ranged from four to more than fifty-one months; and he contended that under the present FDA regulations many drugs now marketed would never have reached clinical trials, including epinephrine, tetracycline, penicillin, cortisone, streptomycin, insulin and—of course—aspirin.

Bad as things were, de Haen reported, they might well become worse with expected new restrictive legislation, the anticipated FDA review of efficacy and safety of non-prescription drugs, and plans to audit prescriptions written by physicians—"Which could result in an unfortunate control of medical practice by the computer."

Eminent statesmen of science in the spring of 1970 had advised Congress that the United States was about to lose its leadership in world science. Some of them thought the country already had become, at best, second-rate. Four who uttered these sobering statements had been advisors to recent presidents: Dr. James R. Killian, then Chairman of the Board of MIT, Dr. Jerome B. Wiesner, MIT Provost, Dr. George B. Kistiakowsky, Professor of Chemistry at Harvard, and Donald F. Hornig, President-elect of Brown. Two others—Dr. Lee A. DuBridge, President Nixon's science advisor, and Handler were of the opinion that the United States already might have forfeited its supremacy.

Handler said, "The heyday of American science could well be behind us for a generation." DuBridge told a symposium, "There has been an upswing in other countries in certain areas, and we are no longer the leader. Maybe we should get used to this idea."

Some felt that the alarms were money-motivated. And, indeed, Handler, a year or two later, said the crisis had passed. Congress and the President had increased their handout to science.

Nevertheless, an extraordinarily opulent nation had come face to face with its god, The Dollar, and found the deity wanting. The United States, which alone spent more on research than all the rest of the countries of the world together and probably an even greater proportion on medicine and medical research, had little to show for its investment. Twelve countries had only a fraction of the infant mortality rate of the United States; in ten others, the citizenry enjoyed a longer life expectancy; and between the two extremes of life, the new American generation was plagued with venereal disease and destroying itself with dope.

Like the gentle rain from heaven, money for many years had fallen on all who had entered research—those in the hard and the soft sciences, M.D.'s, Ph.D.'s, Sc.D.'s, students of the old Mendelian and new molecular genetics, those who probed the atom's interior and those who explored outer space, the geniuses, the workers, the drones, the saints, the fakers, and such alphabetical agencies as NASA, NSF, NIH and FDA. In two or three short decades, science had become the darling, the pet, the fad of American culture. In the American way, armies of scientists were mobilized in crash programs; marble palaces and shining new equipment replaced the smelly old buildings with the creaking floors; rolltop desks on which the mature scientists used to put their feet while they sat in silence and in thought had given way to banks of humming, whistling, pounding, blinking machines spewing out data for fleet-footed young investigators, who had been organized into Task Forces engaged in Team Think. Scientists spent much time at meetings in far reaches of the planet and became authorities on Afghan cookery.

One touch of federal frugality threatened the very foundations of American science. Economy, like money, also had fallen like the gentle rain from heaven—without distinction for intellectual capacity or production of worthwhile ideas, techniques or significant information. The brain drain which had siphoned off many scholars from other lands now flowed the other way—back home. The overlords of science, a singularly undistinguished lot who controlled the funding, were now in command; they could exterminate a thinker or extinguish an idea with a stroke of the pen.

As 1973 begins and this account ends, this is the status of some of the principals of the DMSO story:

Dr. X, whom the FDA had punished in the press and then forgiven, had regained most of his respectability. He had sought support for his research from numerous sources and discovered a private foundation which would finance him.

Grey Keinsley got his master's degree and a job at a bank. His improvement was continuing steadily. At this writing, he can move both legs. A search of the literature discloses no case in which a comparable quadriplegia ever had improved to the degree Grey registered. Jacob said that all but two of the dozen cases of traumatic paraplegia he had treated had shown varying degrees of recovery under DMSO treatment. According to the big battery of neurological tests applied periodically to Grey by a neutral neurologist (hired by Jacob), none of Jacob's other patients had made quite the progress Grey had made—due mainly to the fact that none of the others had so far to go; Grey's treatment began almost two years after his accident and had been interrupted by the FDA ban for about two and one half years; other quadriplegics treated with DMSO soon after their accident made relatively swift and spectacular recoveries.

Harry E. Palmer improved measurably from his nerve blindness, and so did several similar patients. Some of them—those with progressive disease like retinitis pigmentosa—were fortunate enough to have the disease arrested, although it was debatable as to whether the pathologic process was reversed. Nate Amato never did regain any sight, although he continued to experience "flashes"; his aches and pains were well controlled with DMSO. An ophthalmologist associate of Jacob, Dr. Robert V. Hill of the University of Oregon Medical School, treated fifty patients with DMSO for such serious eye diseases as retinitis pigmentosa, macular degeneration and optic atrophy secondary to terminal glaucoma with what he termed "remarkably good results, overall."

Agent 009 insisted that he and the FDA had acted properly in 1965 when they xeroxed Jacob's files and Rosenbaum's records until they were made to leave the premises. He said the call-back of inspectors to Washington for briefing on the DMSO crackdown was not a record (only about fourteen or fifteen inspectors attended the meeting, he said). He said he had no knowledge of Rosenbaum's being induced to sign a blank paper for the FDA ("I know doggone good and well he didn't sign any blank paper for me"). He referred me to the secretary of the Department of Health, Education and Welfare for an answer to Jacob's statement that his personal correspondence had been xeroxed; but he did admit, in effect, that he refused to accede to Jacob's demands for the copies. ("The Xerox rental was paid for by the taxpayers. The Food and Drug pays for it, using their appropriation. The material that goes through the Xerox machine is paid for by the FDA and, in my estimation, is FDA property. Now it was not in my power to do any doggone thing in regard to the material.")

Near the end of our long telephone conversation in Seattle, 009 volunteered: "Frankly, I have great admiration for Dr. Jacob. I don't know how that man does all the work that he does. He's a dynamo! My golly, have you seen his textbook on anatomy? Isn't that a terrific thing? And, holy mackerel, he brought this out while he was doing all that work on DMSO. I think the country is pretty doggone fortunate in having people who have the terrific work capacity and the terrific devotion to their chosen profession so that we can advance the healing arts. And he also tends to his instructional work. I don't know when he gets any sleep."

Commissioner Edwards at this time was still manfully defending the FDA ramparts with all the management expertise at his command. One of the many challenges he faced was a protest to President Nixon by 101 prominent scientists, including Nobelists Salvador Luria, M.D., Julius Axelrod, M.D., and Linus Pauling, Ph.D., against "barriers to research which have been erected deep in the bowels of Federal Bureaucracy." The scientists warned that unless the restraints on responsible researchers were removed, "research will grind slower and slower until it virtually ceases, at a time when it is needed more than ever before."

While Edwards managed to put down all his critics, he did so only by dint of the tremendous range of his oratorical skills and his genius in appealing to almost every human emotion and appetite. Typical of his spellbinding prowess, for example, were his remarks (with his underlining and my headings) at the Fourteenth Annual Meeting of the Pharmaceutical Manufacturers Association:

HUMILITY—I stand before you as the man who at this moment is *sitting* on some 150 NDA's, each of which I should have issued yesterday! I stand before you as a symbol of the power and might of a government which doesn't always hear your voice.

PITY—And lights burn long at night in an Administration that tries and works and then tries again to solve a legacy of staggering problems.

CHARITY—Our prime mission is *not* a *negative* one, dishing out a spectrum of punishment from the wrist slap to the clobber.

REGULATION IS GOOD FOR YOU—A more aggressive administration of regulatory law, backed by more and better science, better protects you, the physician and the public against any charlatan who may spring up in your midst.

FEAR—CONSUMERISM—The consumer movement itself is bringing heavy pressure to bear on both industry and government. This too is here to stay—make no mistake about it!

FEAR: REFORMERISM—There is, of course, a real threat of exactly that—of destructive rather than constructive regulation—for there are those among the new reformers who seemingly will accept nothing short of damage to the industry as evidence of public protection.

FAITH—And *please*, gentlemen, no more nonsense like "aspirin or penicillin could never get FDA approval under present NDA requirements." Now you know that's not so.

HOPE—Now, what are we doing to eliminate the time, cost and delay that plagues new drug applications? We have set up a task force to detect the faults in our internal procedures . . . matched this with a major contract to Auerbach Associates to conduct an extensive study of these same internal FDA procedures . . . we are developing guidelines for clinical research . . . planning new strategies for sorting out IND's . . . soliciting new ideas. . . .

LOVE (FAMILY)—Fifteen hundred new drug products were marketed in one foreign country in 1970, and it was reported that 90 per cent of these could not be prescribed in the United States. But which country's drug laws would you choose for *your* family?

LOVE (COUNTRY)—The FDA can not abdicate its responsibility to the *American* public in favor of some similar body abroad.

CENSORSHIP—We at FDA are interested in helping you move to promotion more legitimately educational in nature. The present guidelines for advertising must be reviewed and revised.

SHUT UP—I suggest to you that we avoid the needless confrontation which only dissipates our resources and yours while delivering no benefit to the public.

This very well may have been the silver-tongued commissioner's finest display of management expertise. It mattered not that many of his statements seemed a brazen contradiction of the experts' data, or that his new task forces probably would repeat the

355

relatively recent jobs done by the Ritts and Kinslow committees, or that he was glossing over, with euphemisms, complaints that the citizenry were losing their basic liberties to an ever more intrusive bureaucracy. The things he said, and how he said them, and the things he left unsaid could be understood by his audience, an industrial association which had welcomed into its opulent ranks so many retired FDA officers and which, in all likelihood, would continue this generous practice.

Outside the hall in Boca Raton, Florida, where Edwards spoke, the natives were becoming restless. Throughout the land some concerned citizens were beginning to murmur against mammoth corporations and trade associations which, they contended, were buying up their government and their civil rights.

In the spring of 1973, the FDA was facing a familiar situation —a series of imminent disasters. Scientists were petitioning for reforms which might bring a measure of freedom and honesty back to research and help American science and medicine regain a measure of its former prestige. Paul de Haen's new authoritative *Drug Products Parade* was showing with data that could not be dismissed that in 1972 America had made another giant step toward pharmacological and medical oblivion in an increasingly competitive world. An unsympathetic press was calling attention to unrestricted carcinogens, teratogens and other toxins and filth in food; the AP carried a story quoting an independent research organization as stating that sodium nitrite, a color preservative in meat, was making bacon and hot dogs "the most dangerous food in the supermarket" from a cancer-causing viewpoint. And there were the usual demands that the FDA be abolished and replaced with something workable.

Edwards, keeping his cool, parried all these thrusts. He issued a stream of press releases calling attention to new crises and diverting attention from FDA critics. The FDA announced the recall of hundreds of thousands of cans of a product because one was found botulism-tainted (nobody hurt); it called for labeling that would disclose the amount of real orange juice in supermarket orange juice and offered "government-approved" labels to producers who behaved themselves (many thought this was also a ploy in the FDA's old war to restrict vitamins and essential mineral fortification from foods); it secured indictments for contaminated intravenous fluids; it proposed changes in labeling and advertising claims for some antacids; it admonished drug houses to prove that their antibiotic and other additives in cattle feeds (which often wind up in the system of meat eaters) were safe; it warned doctors against falsifying data; it even approved an IND for gerovital, or H-3, a Rumanian preparation which allegedly ameliorated many of the major symptoms and diseases of aging—a reversal of its twenty-five-year opposition.

Edwards told a Senate subcommittee, "We are proud of the fact that, while the public has been deprived of no significant drugs, we have been able to achieve and maintain the best safety record of any drug-producing nation in the world." For dramatic emphasis, he had an aide, Dr. Henry E. Simmons tell again the oft-told tale of thalidomide and explain that Americans need not go abroad for any kind of safe and sane drug treatment. The latter was in response to the assertion by a UCLA economist, Sam Peltzman, that the thalidomide panic, in terms of money, morbidity and mortality, had inspired a delay in drug introductions from ten to a hundred times as costly as the teratogenic debacle itself.

The FDA's many-sided mouth, Edwards' broken field talking, the double and triple reverses, the finesse with which nosy newsmen could be taken out of a play, the sportsmanlike camaraderie with the opposing drug houses—these did not escape notice.

Scouts from the highest echelon were impressed with the FDA's team and its super-manager. The White House inner circle—the varsity squad—had been blundering from one bad situation to a worse one: The coaches were going to jail for burglary and bugging; some of the stars were proving themselves liars; the election gamblers, it appeared, had become the private owners

357

and operators of the team, and once again the press was kicking around the captain.

So President Nixon reached into the farm club and recruited its star. He appointed Edwards HEW assistant secretary for health, which gave him control not only of the FDA but also of every health agency in the department.

One of Edwards' initial challenges was to make PSRO operative. PSRO, or Professional Standards Review Organization, presumably was a self-policing system established by an act of Congress and signature of the President for the medical profession. Ostensibly it was designed to weed out incompetent doctors; however, some feared that because of the innate faults of the peer review system and the financial control wielded over it by a tough bureaucracy, medical incompetence might come to include scientific concepts contrary to those of the bureau and dangerous—subversive, that is—attitudes toward the administration. This was an area not entirely unfamiliar to the FDA.

Of the PSRO program, Edwards said: "It's going to demand an unbelievable degree of cooperation between the public and private sectors of medicine—a degree beyond any I've ever seen, and this includes organized medicine." At the same time, social security and medical records were being made available to inspection by departmental police; and while this breach of confidentiality might make it easier to catch cheaters, it also brought a new degree of Big Brotherism into the American government. The citizens' most intimate secrets—their health histories, their use of medical-care systems, and their financial status—became available to bureaucracy's in-group.

It also fell to Edwards to preside over and explain the administration's junking national health programs and cutting back sharply quotas for university faculties and the training of new scientists and doctors. Economy was given as the reason, but Edwards was hard put to find a silver lining in the situation.

While Edwards went onward and upward, Goddard, who had dropped completely out of the news when he resigned five years earlier, became visible again. Items in the paramedical press announced that the former FDA commissioner had three appointments: 1) chairman of the Medical Advisory Committee of Somatronics, Inc., a developer and distributor of x-ray and other medical electronic equipment, 2) Board Chairman of Ormont Drug & Chemical Co., and 3) consultant to Diagnostic Data, Inc., a pharmaceutical and development firm based in California. Goddard had spent some time in India. He had let his crewcut grow almost to shoulder length, and his once angular, cleanshaven features now were wreathed in a flowing beard.

Hodges, the aide who had sat in with Goddard during our interview, had followed Sadusk in retirement; he became a vice president of the Detroit drug house, Parke, Davis & Co.; he was in charge of research and development, and in press releases he was proclaiming the merits of his employer's synthetic skin and other products.

Sadusk, meanwhile, had become senior vice-president of the parent company, Warner Lambert, and was now railing at his old employer, the FDA. At a Clinical Pharmacological Methods Symposium in 1973, he placed on view 456 volumes, totaling 1.5 tons of data, on one New Drug Application for a simple muscle relaxant. He complained that it takes from five to more than fourteen years, with an outlay of many millions of dollars, to introduce a new drug onto the market. He deplored the threat of criminal liability for erroneous data. The FDA shoe, now on the other foot, pinched.

Frances Lorraine Ames, who had been denied the benefits of DMSO for so many years, finally found release from the terrible pains. Death, the supreme analgesic, set her free in 1972.

And Sidney Farber followed his onetime associate, Morris Green, down the dusty road to destiny. It was his battered heart which did him in early in the eventful spring of 1973. In his life, he had done a great deal for the cancer ill of the world. In death, he had left much undone.

Almost six years after the FDA ban on DMSO, American physicians were as ignorant as ever of the drug's safety and efficacy record. DMSO's curious effects on mouse cancer viruses in American research seemed to go unnoticed, along with DMSO's prevention of kidney stones in rats in experiments at Hospital Richat in Paris, or the success and enthusiasm of scientists in Estonian research centers who had found DMSO effective against a spectrum of serious infections associated with surgery.

The tragedy of ignorance is reflected in the experience of a forty-year-old woman neighbor of ours who, after two years of presenting her puzzling symptoms to one physician after another, finally had been diagnosed as having scleroderma. Concerned almost to the point of panic and herself a practicing psychologist, she consulted all the standard references and came to the conclusion that medicine had very little to offer her. Her physicians prescribed physical therapy three times a week and enough thorazine to keep her in an almost perpetual stupor. I suggested she ask her doctors about DMSO. She did. "One of them laughed uproariously," she told me. "The other one asked me, 'Do you want to go blind too?' I went to another specialist in another hospital—a neurologist who was getting a big grant for research on scleroderma. He said, 'There are thirty drugs like DMSO—all of them no good. DMSO would give you cataracts.' " The doctor told her bluntly, and perhaps brutally, that there was nothing that would help her. Nevertheless, he prescribed potassium p-aminobenzoate and sent her home. The doctors declined to review the New York Academy proceedings. At this writing, there are numerous ulcers on our friend's fingers; her face is masklike; her skin has turned to leather. She has trouble swallowing.

The FDA by banning research with DMSO (except sporadically, in a few patients and a few centers) has: 1) deprived people in pain of its blessings; 2) discouraged animal and human experiments which would disclose all the conditions for which it is indicated; and 3) made it impossible to determine the true toxicity of DMSO, and this may be the greatest disservice of all. While there seems to be not the slightest credible laboratory or clinical evidence of DMSO's harming human beings, every knowledgeable scientist who has worked with DMSO stands in awe of its theoretical potential for injury as well as its great good. We do not know, for instance, what DMSO might do to a baby bathed with soap containing high levels of hexachlorophene, the deodorant suspected of having killed some infants by its action on the brain and peripheral nerves. In this case, would the DMSO exercise an additive, synergistic, detoxifying or completely negligible influence on the hexachlorophene? The FDA's actions have discouraged efforts to determine what effect DMSO will have in concert with perhaps hundreds of other common chemicals in our environment—drugs, cosmetics, food, and pollutants of all sorts. It seems unlikely that the FDA can discourage patients forever with fairy tales of DMSO's alleged toxicity or by suppressing the established facts of its therapeutic merit.

Bob Herschler had no regular employment after Crown Zellerbach fired him. Herschler's refusal to communicate with Jacob for more than three years (at Crown's insistence, he said) apparently had left no lasting scar. Jacob dipped into his own meager funds to pay Herschler $200 a month to work on the bibliography of Jacob's forthcoming book *Dimethyl Sulfoxide, Vol. II,* which will be the definitive work on clinical applications of DMSO; the book will be brought out by Marcel Dekker, Inc., possibly late in 1974. Jacob is making Herschler a co-author.

When I visited with Herschler in Portland in October 1972, he had been spending a good deal of time planning the synthesis of new compounds. He felt that he could attach a lipophilic group of atoms to the DMSO molecule which would clear the bloodstream and, hopefully, arterial walls of cholesterol and other lipids which some authorities hold responsible for hardened arteries and the diseases they give rise to. He also believed he could produce DMSO from petroleum products cheaper than it was now being synthesized from lignin. In an era of inflation, he might reduce the basic price of a fair grade of DMSO to twenty or twenty-five cents a pound (or a pint) and of top medical grade DMSO to about twice that figure, he thought. And even if the markup were ten or a hundred times the cost of the raw product, DMSO still stood to be the cheapest and most useful product on drugstore shelves.

Herschler felt that one of DMSO's greatest uses would be in agriculture, the field in which he first had tested it. He said that eight pounds of it distributed over an acre would increase the yield—of corn, for example—between 10 and 30 per cent. He said that when Crown fired him he was experimenting with DMSO combined with pesticides; he felt that the right combinations could be substituted for DDT-type poisons and greatly reduce this kind of pollution of the environment.

One or two foundations seemed to be seriously considering supporting Herschler's research; and this could be a godsend. It might be many years, if ever, until royalties, with or without court intervention, would become available for the space, the equipment, the animals and the help for a productive laboratory.

In the spring of 1973, Henry D. Moyle, Jr., president of Research Industries Corporation, a small but vigorous conglomerate headquartered in Salt Lake City, told me he was seeking a chemist to synthesize DMSO from oil for him. Moyle was contemplating establishing outpatient clinics specializing in DMSO treatments in Mexico.

In countries which had ignored as best they could the FDA's alarums, DMSO still was not a profitable product. The FDA's refusal to countenance the great therapeutic effects of the drug and the FDA's unsubstantiated insinuations of toxicity deterred drug houses abroad from promoting DMSO. The FDA seemed hung up on the hope that DMSO would turn out to be another thalidomide and thus vindicate its early panic-producing actions. Dr. Gerhard Laudahn, Director of Schering AG in Berlin, had written me earlier that he had not promoted his DMSO, despite the fact that "I consider DMSO to be an extremely promising drug with a large range of application. I believe it to be one of the major discoveries of our time." Germany too was thalidomide-conscious and heeded the FDA.

Nicolas Weinstein and the Chilean scientists who had reported such signal success of DMSO mixtures against a dictionary of diseases were not overly impressed by American bureaucracy, so they conducted many controlled tests and came up with a rosy picture of DMSO's performance. The United States sent a couple of investigators down to Chile to look over the situation; their first report was a splendid example of bureaucratic gobbledegoop in that it said nothing good, nothing bad, nothing at all that they could be pinned down on about the work they (a representative of the FDA and another of the National Institute of Mental Health) had seen. Stanley Jacob, who arranged the itinerary and escorted them, had some of Chile's finest scientists, physicians and others discuss their work, show their publications, supply reprints, and answer questions. In their report, the commission—as it was called—almost got Jacob's name right; they spelled it Jacobs. They had little or nothing to say about the retarded children whose minds had been greatly improved with DMSO, nor the oldsters whose arteries to the heart and brain had been reopened, nor any of the many other DMSO effects which had been demonstrated.

Ed Rosenbaum and Stanley Jacob did not meet often any more. Once DMSO had established itself—legally abroad and extralegally here—as an agent of awesome therapeutic uses, there no longer was need for this close working relationship. With the threats and the pressures off, each member of this mismatched pair gravitated back to his chosen way of life. Rosenbaum occupied himself with his thriving practice and pleasant home life—Jacob with his professional obsessions, and Sundays with his sons.

Don Wood, the biochemist who worked closely with Jacob, felt that DMSO's most useful roles in medicine were yet to come to light. He believed that DMSO as dilute as 4 or 5 per cent, given by routes other than on the skin, would prove effective in many therapies. These, he said, are the concentrations in which strong DMSO reaches the bloodstream when topically applied. He regarded DMSO's remarkable ability to dissolve a wide range of biological compounds—like cholesterol, cholesterol esters, collagen and some enzymes—as opening the door to new treatments of heart and vascular conditions, and some of the symptoms of aging. He cited 90 per cent DMSO's ability to dissolve hematomas, like the strawberry birthmark, within minutes, while 20 per cent DMSO will be without effect; such factors as concentration, he said, incite disputes over the drug's often contrary effects. He believes the brightest promise of all lies in DMSO's tendency to add to or multiply the therapeutic effects of other agents and to detoxify still others. Early in 1973, Wood accepted a job with a chemical house in his native Salt Lake City to be near his family.

The environment of Stanley Jacob included patients and physicians, bureaucrats and politicians, creditors and supporters (the latter being mainly Uncle Morris). And then there were serendipity and empiricism to fascinate him and critics to moor him to reality.

Jacob had a patient with peptic ulcer and considerably elevated systolic and diastolic heartbeat pressures, none of which was responding to conventional treatment. The patient asked for DMSO to apply to his skin for lumbosacral pains. Within a week all symptoms relented; the patient was almost normal. Jacob found that the patient, on his own, had been taking a shot of DMSO in orange juice daily, and this gave his critics new fodder. Jacob felt that the anti-ulcer effects tended to confirm the French claims that very weak oral doses of DMSO were good for many things that ail the digestive tract.

For the most part, however, Jacob concentrated on the kind of conditions for which neither DMSO nor any other treatment wrought instant miracle cures—the most challenging diseases that he had encountered during a decade of experimentation in almost 5,000 patients. Traumatic paraplegia was one (with ten out of twelve patients improved during periods up to fifty-four months), nerve blindness (like macular degeneration, traumatic blindness, retinitis pigmentosa and the like), stroke (his dozen stroke patients had made enough progress to encourage him to explore the field), mental retardation (with improvement in four out of every five cases, including mongolism), and emphysema (only two cases but both yielding good symptomatic and objective results).

There was the steady stream of reprints from abroad to buttress his faith (which needed no strengthening). Like the paper by Dr. Elfren Solano Aguilar of the University of Costa Rica, who reported excellent results of DMSO (mixed with triamcinolone) against several kinds of dermatitis—atopic, contact, seborrheic, actinic, varicose and neural) but with good, bad and indifferent results with psoriasis and acne vulgaris. T. Szydlowska and others of Lodz, Poland, confirmed the observations of Charles E. Huggins of Harvard that DMSO preserves cells for long periods; the Polish scientist also showed that DMSO made some normally resistant bacteria vulnerable to antibiotic attack.

Scientists at Cambridge University reported that "surrogate motherhood" had crossed the line from science fiction to scientific fact, thanks to the coolant properties of DMSO. They had: 1) removed the ten-day fertilized ovum from the uterus of Cow A; 2) treated it with DMSO (which displaced some of the cells' water) and stored it for six days at minus 169° C; 3) rewarmed it slowly and implanted it in the uterus of Cow B, where it developed normally and eventually was delivered as a healthy bull calf. The scientists viewed the procedure as a means of maintaining genetic banks and incubating in ordinary animals until birth the early embryos of quality males and females. Another possibility is for women volunteers to nurture through pregnancy and bear the offspring of couples who for some reason need this help. Scientists at the Oak Ridge National Laboratory in Tennessee are co-operating with the Cambridge group.

A few new researchers entered the DMSO picture in the United States, undaunted by the formidable FDA barriers. Foremost among them was Jack C. de la Torre, Ph.D., Sc.D., Assistant Professor of Neurosurgery at the University of Chicago, who simulated in laboratory animals the head and spinal cord injuries which kill many thousand Americans every year in traffic accidents; the DMSO-treated animals survived far better and recovered much sooner than controls.

Much as he detested it, money had continued to be Jacob's most pressing problem. Betty Lou King, the Portland socialite who reviewed with Jacob the Chilean work with retarded children, organized a "Ziegfeld Years" show which played to a capacity audience and netted $15,000 for DMSO research. Her son, Billy, continued along the long road back toward normality; his tongue no longer protruded; he had achieved bladder and bowel control; his vocabulary had increased from zero to 300 words. A few patients and a few well-wishers donated to DMSO research. Jacob maintained his amateur standing by getting a loan on the Oldsmobile that Jack Brandis, his cancer patient, had insisted on giving him, and he turned the money over to DMSO research. The net effect of Brandis's generosity was, for Jacob, a more reliable car and another sizable bill to pay each month.

New sources of funds for research seemed to be opening up. The Clipped Wings—the society of airline stewardesses who had married and retired—invited Jacob to talk about his work with retarded children; and after his lecture they gave the DMSO foundation a check for $8,700. A society interested in retinitis pigmentosa began inquiring into his work in that disease. And a young and independent drug house began negotiating for data that Squibb had collected and shelved. The majority stock holder of the new company was impressed by DMSO and determined to put it on the market if the deal could be made.

Crown collected its first royalties ($12,000) from Syntex for veterinary DMSO used on horses. At this writing the money remains in Crown's custody.

With no fanfare, without so much as a news release or a proud proclamation by Commissioner Edwards, the FDA quietly—almost furtively—extended to dogs the limited benefits of DMSO that it earlier had given horses. Three announcements buried in the Federal Registers were circulated among nineteen officials of the FDA. On May 25, 1972, the notice said DMSO could be given topically to reduce swelling due to trauma in dogs (20 ml per day for fourteen days) and in horses (100 ml per day for thirty days, maximum). Excluded were animals intended for breeding and horses to be slaughtered for food. The DMSO was for use only by or on the order of a licensed veterinarian. On July 20, a notice stated that fa/DMSO (0.01 per cent fluocinolone acetonide in 60 per cent DMSO with propylene glycol and citric acid) could be instilled in a dog's ear twice a day for fourteen days in treatment of the itching and inflammation of acute and chronic otitis. On August 25, the Register announced that fa/DMSO could be used to treat inflammation and impaction of the anal sac, commonly called the "stink gland," in dogs.

Ten years, more than 1,200 scientific papers, and perhaps more than a million patients—human patients, that is—after the first clinical experiments with DMSO, Commissioner Edwards and his brain trust had permitted its use in the dog ear and anus.

Well, it was progress.

In Jacob's care, Jack Brandis outlived his expectancy (originally set at one week) by more than six months, thanks to bold therapeutic quarterbacking. When one treatment began to lose its power to arrest the disease, another was substituted. Brandis became the beneficiary of a long series of incomplete remissions, which afforded him good days and bad. On Thanksgiving Day, he was well enough to enjoy having his family, including his eight grandchildren, with him. Early the next morning the cancer overwhelmed temperature and respiratory control centers of his brain; and he went to sleep quietly and courageously slipped out of a life which had provided him so extravagantly with its bounty.

Brandis's friends contributed almost $20,000 to the DMSO Research Fund "in lieu of flowers."

A few months later, friends of the legendary Frank Leahy were asked to contribute to the DMSO Research Fund "in lieu of flowers." Jacob had treated the football coaching immortal for an agonizing arthritis during the five years that Leahy fought a losing battle with leukemia.

Thalidomide, the teratogen which had produced about 10,000 grotesquely crippled infants and which inadvertently had contributed to the DMSO debacle, appeared to be making a comeback of sorts. Dr. Joseph Sheskin of Hadassah University Hospital, Jerusalem, tested it against leprosy's most fearful consequences, the "lepra reaction" marked by high fever, excruciating pain of joints and muscles, and ugly eruptions; thalidomide rapidly and completely reversed the symptoms in 90 per cent of the cases and sedated the patients without, however, affecting the underlying leprosy to any curative degree. Thalidomide is being tested against other puzzling conditions, with careful avoidance of use in pregnant women.

The story of Stanley Jacob and DMSO and the FDA is not new. It is as old as science and medicine are old. Only the names are new; the rest is a plagiarism that dates back to man's first fascination with the firmament, his first efforts to understand and heal the life within and about him.

Four centuries before Christ, Hippocrates took issue with the convention of treating a fever by inducing a chill (which killed the patient), and he implored his devoted students to place their patients' welfare above all, and "if there be an opportunity of serving one who is a stranger in financial straits, give full assistance to all such."

Like Jacob, Archimedes had an excess of enthusiasm. When, on conceiving the principle of specific gravity, he leaped out of his tub and ran naked through the streets of Syracuse, Sicily, shouting, "Eureka!"—which means "I have found it!" He too lacked the abject attitude authorities like; at seventy-five, Archimedes sat in the street drawing diagrams in the dust when an invading Roman soldier got in his way; when Archimedes asked the soldier to move, the Roman naturally drew his sword and ran the old man through. Merely enforcing the law.

Roger Bacon, the monk, frittered away his time making lenses while the right-thinking bureaucrats and alchemists called his dreams of building flying carriages and producing living quarters under the sea black magic and the work of the devil. The rebellious and unrepentant Bacon spent fourteen years in prison.

Galileo Galilei, the Pisa professor of mathematics, was cursed with the weakness of blurting out the truth as he saw it. Copernicus, the Prussian-born Polish priest-doctor, disputed—but discreetly—the Church-approved doctrine of Ptolemy that Earth was the center of where the celestial action was . . . not the sun. The Establishment, even in that day, was inclined to brook no doubts. Copernicus prudently kept his theories on paper until shortly before his death, when he published them, with an inserted apology to the Pope. Headstrong Galileo, on the other hand, uttered his heresies; he went blind after staring at the sun.

Leonardo da Vinci, 500 years ago, let the world revere him for his art, but he dared not discuss his scientific achievements. It was only when he was safely in his grave that the testament that he had roughed out, in secret code, disclosed his principles of tunnel-boring and canal-cutting devices, airplanes, steam propulsion, paddle wheels, explosives and bullets and many other incredible concepts. He dissected bodies, drew remarkably accurate pictures of tissues, organs and systems. The work could have been the first great anatomy textbook. He had worked out a fine classification of the animal kingdom, but, because his contemporaries were not ready for it, he left to a later generation—Galileo, Copernicus and Lamarck—the glory and the abuse of publishing. The Austrian monk Gregor Mendel was restrained, self-effacing; and his observations on genetics, which revolutionized biological sciences, were lost for fifty years as a result.

Stanley Jacob's mother once told me about the time her son came home with "the only bad grade he ever received—a B-plus in swimming during his high school sophomore year." He blurted out the news and bawled. He did not get over his heartbreak at once. For years, his mother said, he was haunted by a fear of failure, although his grades never again went lower than A's.

A small sense of insecurity hung over Jacob as he sat in the Lecture Room waiting to be summoned into the Board Room of the National Academy of Sciences to tell the *ad hoc* Committee on DMSO his views. The committee had invited him, along with others, to appear on this early spring morning in 1973 and provide "such new scientific information on DMSO, or references thereto, which might have escaped the Committee's survey." The NAS/NRC's long investigation was due to wind up within the next couple of months; the findings would be passed along to the FDA, which was financing the study, and presumably the FDA would report the results in a manner consistent with the wishes of its officials and its press agents.

The uneasiness Jacob felt as he reread for the seventh time the tenth draft of the statement he had prepared for the committee was largely intuitive—supported in the main by memories of the FDA's attacks upon him, his associates, his beloved DMSO.

370

He had not heard as yet of the report "Nader's Raiders" were soon to release which would impugn the integrity of NAS/NRC committees, like the one now about to determine the fate of DMSO. Philip M. Boffey, a science writer associate of Ralph Nader, had discovered, during a two-year investigation of the NAS, that members of the powerful advisory panels had promoted some commercial products and concealed evidence against others in abiding by the wishes of the federal officers whose agencies financed their studies. It seemed unlikely that the *ad hoc* DMSO Committee could make the FDA, its creator, happy with a report indicating that the FDA had committed another enormous error in banning DMSO for eight long years.

Jacob was acutely aware of the degeneration which was rotting the political and governmental processes of his country. He had been a victim during the early phases of the disease which now had become epidemic. He was familiar with the "no-knock" system, the photocopying of private papers, bugging, punitive investigations, slander and libel, character assassination, forgery, lying and blackmail.

The trend in the technology of applied political science had been progressively toward more sophisticated practices, as the news media now were reporting. No-knock, for example, was being practiced by thirty-eight teams of agents of the Bureau of Narcotics and Dangerous Drugs, originally an FDA creation which had been turned over to the Department of Justice; the teams, tough, heavily armed, profane, violent, sometimes in parties resembling hippie motorcycle gangs, were terrorizing innocent communities as well as narcotic rings.

The "Watergate investigation" was bringing to light a new lexicon: lying statements were excused as being "no longer operative"; written words were run through the shredding machines or "deep-sixed"; critical citizens were named on enemy lists to be subjected to electronic bugging, burglary, tax audits, harassment by several government agencies and other measures of "internal security." Members of all social and professional groups

371

and in all communities were being enlisted to spy upon their neighbors for "informer fees." The creators and managers of the systems were paid with tax dollars and given immunity under "executive privilege."

Stanley Jacob was determined that DMSO would not be denied because of the hostility of his critics, the conventions of conformity of his profession, the rapacity of an industry and venality of a calling which feeds upon the suffering of the sick and the dying, the brutality of a political system undergoing malignant transformation, and certainly not because of his own timidity. On March 9, 1973, he appeared before the NAS/NRC ad hoc committee studying the DMSO matter and said:

> Historically, a new therapeutic principle is often difficult to accept. The concept purporting "one drug, one medical application" is disproved by the challenge of the DMSO principle. In my opinion, no physician, unless he has treated patients with DMSO, particularly those refractory to conventional therapy, can grasp the inherent therapeutic value.
>
> Since beginning evaluations of DMSO in 1963, I have seen a wide spectrum of diseases respond favorably. I have not seen a single serious side effect; the beneficial effects in diseases, many refractory to other therapy, have been observed and reported upon by numbers of physicians, most unknown to me and practicing in many parts of the world.
>
> DMSO comes closer than any chemical with which I am familiar to filling a real medical need for the majority of their life-sustaining animals and even their food crops.

Jacob predicted that DMSO, when injected alone or in combination with other drugs, would prove useful against many common cripplers and killers—acute injuries to the brain and nervous system, cancers, blindness, stroke and paraplegias. He said it soon could be obtained from a variety of sources for twenty or thirty cents a pint—"a price afforded by a majority of citizens of the world."